FRONT DESK SECRETS

of the Nation's Fastest Growing Orthodontic Practices

Luke Infinger

Front Desk Secrets of the Nation's Fastest Growing Orthodontic Practices

ISBN-13: 978-1-990476-05-1

Published by: Expert Author Press
https://www.expertauthorpress.com/

Canadian Address:
1908 – 1251 Cardero Street,
Vancouver, BC, Canada, V6G 2H9
Phone: (604) 941-3041
info@expertauthorpress.com

A Note From The Author

As humans, we typically complicate most things.

You've probably heard of the KISS principle: "Keep it simple stupid." Over the years, I have seen that applying this principle to business increases efficiency, productivity, and profit. I bring this up because many of you may read this book and think, "It can't be that simple... "Do you mean if we just call the leads quickly... text them right away...then we will get more starts?" Well, to be honest, it is a little more complicated than that. But not by much! That's why I wrote this book.

It all starts with having the right people. You can actually throw experience out of the window. If your scheduling team doesn't have the right PERSONALITY and the right MINDSET, it just won't work. Think back to a bad customer service experience you had, maybe even at a doctor's office. Was the front desk exceptional? Were you contacted quickly? At check-in, was there a frosted glass window separating you from a standoffish team member who said as little as possible in a monotone voice? Did you have to wait longer than five or ten minutes to be called back?

Now, think back to a great experience. Maybe it was at Chick-fil-A, Starbucks, The Ritz, or a local business. What made the experience great? Was the first touch a

WOW? Someone probably stood out on both occasions. Attitude and mindset make a HUGE difference. In this book, I explain why you are costing yourself thousands of dollars each day by:

- Not hiring the right people for your front desk.
- Not having daily statistics on your scheduling team.
- Not setting scheduling goals.
- Not giving your team incentives to hit those goals.

Leaving your team's training to chance and hoping for the best.

Several of the nation's fastest-growing orthodontic practices have been completely transformed by the procedures and scripts I share in this book. You'll hear about breakthroughs that orthodontists just like you have had by shifting their mindset on their front desk and the vital role of their schedulers.

I invite you to share this book with your office manager and team. I hope it inspires and challenges you to apply the principles. And please, reach out and share how things change in your practice.

Best,

Luke Infinger
Co-Founder & CEO at HIP

Special Thanks

A number of people made contributions to this book which, in my humble opinion, have made it much more engaging and easy to read. Thank you to Fishbein Orthodontics for their visionary leadership within the profession; to Amanda Floyd, the COO, who inspires team members everywhere to lead with clarity and purpose; and to Alyx Perry, the Director of Patient Communications, who lifts scheduling coordinators to new heights with her positivity.

I am ever grateful for Beverly Simkins, the Lead Front Desk Coordinator at Cassinelli, Shanker, & Baker, who truly loves her role and enjoys serving each new patient. And a huge thanks to Julie Zhur, a Location Manager and Front Office Training Specialist at Sunrise Orthodontics, who has a wealth of knowledge and expertise.

I am very grateful to Harrison Bagdan, the Senior Practice Advisor at HIP, for his dedication, passion, and commitment to scheduling coordinators everywhere.

Thank you all for being the inspiration for this book and maintaining a standard that makes me proud and excited to keep learning and making HIP's education better than ever before!

TABLE OF CONTENTS

Introduction

As the first quarter of 2022 was winding down and I was putting the final touches on this manuscript, it struck me how quickly the world is shifting. After two years of a global pandemic transforming the face of business forever, I realized that thriving in the new reality means embracing the ever-accelerating pace of change. Success in this new world requires business owners to constantly adapt to the ever-changing preferences of the customer. The Amazon-inspired, instant gratification, "click and get right away" culture has reshaped every business.

When a lead fills out a web form for a complimentary orthodontic consultation, they want a response right away. If a scheduling coordinator calls them within five minutes, that lead can be converted to a new patient, adding $5,000.00 or $6,000.00 to the practice. However, if the front desk operates like the industry average, that scheduling coordinator probably won't call that lead back until two days later, and by that point, they will have scheduled their consultation somewhere else (or worse, go with a DIY aligner company). If your front desk misses just one call a day, that could be costing your practice $1,000,000.00 a year. This is why I consider the scheduling coordinator to be the MOST important role in your clinic. It's also the most overlooked. It's the reason why I wrote a whole book about the front desk secrets that make the nation's fastest-growing orthodontic practices as successful as they are.

Since 2014, I've been studying the business of orthodontics. My company, HIP, has analyzed over a thousand of the fifty-seven hundred independent orthodontic practices in the U.S. and followed consumer behavior trends behind creating great smiles. We have had the privilege of helping some of the fastest-growing practices meet and often exceed their goals. While these practices varied greatly, the common thread was that the orthodontist had a vision for how they wanted to serve their community, a plan for making it real, and metrics that showed them where they were on the path towards their goal. Most importantly, these doctors realized that they had a business to run and that their technical skills generated the most revenue when serving patients.

I have noticed that the medical field's mindset is stuck in the old world view where "people should listen to me because I'm the doctor." People equated the 'doctor' title with some kind of revered sage whose word was not to be questioned. Back then, you were set for life when you beat out all the other people fighting for the privilege of spending hundreds of thousands of dollars and years of their lives to gain that title. Today, orthodontic services are perceived as commodities, and people are shopping around. The impact on orthodontists with the old world mindset has been debilitating.

As a solo orthodontist twenty years ago, you used to be able to open a boutique practice with a team of five or six people and do about $3,000,000.00 in production. A few years ago, I was at a conference and I talked to this guy who started precisely this way. He had built a lifestyle around how his practice used to be. Over the years, his production steadily declined to the point where he was just shy of a million dollars. When he should have been reaping the rewards of all his hard work, he struggled to pay bills and maintain the quality of life that his family had become accustomed to living.

The average orthodontic practice is doing about $1,200,000.00 a year in production. In today's world, that's not a whole lot of money. The chips stack up fast when you come out of residency with $800,000.00 in debt. The insurance game has changed, and the government constantly changes the rules. You've got payroll and taxes, and on top of all that financial stress, there's life: raising a family, paying the mortgage, and building that dream lifestyle you thought you were guaranteed when you got into the profession. It's no wonder the divorce rate is through the roof, and suicides are rising. How do you make this work?

There is just so much competition today, and without question, you have to do marketing to succeed. There are tons of marketing companies who are happy to step in and generate leads for your practice. Ultimately, orthodontists do want the magic solution that will provide them with the steady stream of new patients and starts that they need to create the practice and lifestyle they desire.

At the conference, the guy I talked to was pulling his hair out, trying to figure out what he was doing wrong. Sadly, he was so rooted in the old world mindset that he kept trying to solve the problem on his own. He thought he could save money by trying to run the business himself. He did not realize that there is a massive cost to trying to be the orthodontist and the chief of operations at the same time, and the people who try this end up doing both poorly.

On the flip side, Dr. Ben Fishbein of Fishbein Orthodontics has one of the fastest growing orthodontic practices in the country. Since he partnered with HIP back in 2015, he has grown from three locations and twenty-five team members to eight locations and over one hundred team members. To his credit, Dr. Fishbein always thought more like a business owner than an orthodontist, and he had a clear vision of the business he wanted to build. We created the Patient Acquisition and Retention Framework™ (PARF™) through our partnership with him. You can discover more about this framework in our first book, "The Ultimate Practice–What Medical School Forgot to Teach You About Building the Life of Your Dreams." I'll gladly send you a copy if you reach out to me. At that time, we applied the PARF™ to all sorts of medical practices with excellent results. We have since decided to specialize in the growth of orthodontic practices only.

Scan this QR code to find our first book on Amazon.

Dr. Fishbein had it figured out. He realized that we were flushing marketing dollars down the drain if we just did marketing to generate leads without a system for converting them into patients, wowing them, and retaining them. As his partner, we helped train his team in this framework alongside the marketing campaigns we ran to build a lead conversion machine that has not stopped growing since.

I wrote this book to share what we've learned about growing orthodontic practices, and to help orthodontists build a lifestyle that allows them to serve their community at the level they want while still having time to spend with their families. You may or may not want to grow a multi-location orthodontic practice, but I'm sure you have some vision for the life you want to create. If you have decided that you want to take a leadership role, plan how to realize that vision, and share it with your team, this book is for you. If not, that's okay, too. Whether you have just graduated or have been in the field for twenty years or more, if you want to grow from a boutique practice into a real business, you're looking to take on an associate, or you're thinking of expanding another location, pay close attention.

This book is the first in the four-part "Orthodontic Practice Growth Series." I created this series to compile everything I've learned from working with the fastest-growing orthodontic practices in the nation. Book 1 is about the front desk and the most undervalued role in the practice: the scheduling coordinator. Book 2 will cover the role of the treatment coordinator. Book 3 discusses the importance of having a Chief Operations Officer (COO) in your practice that is not you. Finally, Book 4 will explore the future of orthodontics. While this first book was written with orthodontists in mind, I hope you will share it with your office manager, team leader, and anyone else who wants to grow with the vision you have for your practice. It will take someone else (manager, team lead, etc.) to work with your team to implement the information and process.

Dr. Ben Fishbein didn't start out like this. Listen to what his COO, Amanda Floyd, has to say about his beginnings:

> *"I was the treatment coordinator when Dr. Ben bought the practice. The practice was what they call a boutique practice in the industry. We had one small location that was open three days a week. We saw about thirty patients and four new patients a day. We did two-hour consults, a totally different process from what we do now.*
>
> *We kept everything the same for about a year. Shortly after he bought the practice, I started managing it. He had a five-year goal involving seeing patients and*

someone else overseeing all the processes necessary for that kind of growth. We set out a business plan, and just kind of took it step-by-step. We reached our five-year goal in about a year and a half. Now we're on track this year to quadruple."

To emphasize what's possible, Dr. Fishbein was so clear on his vision for the practice that he and his team were able to put systems in place to reduce the time spent in a new patient consult from two hours to one minute. A change like that does not happen overnight, and to be clear, the patient still gets a WOW experience from all team members involved in the process.

Here's what Amanda has to say about transforming their practice:

"We did it in increments, honestly. We started at two hours, and then we shortened it to an hour and a half, and then to an hour. Then we shortened it to forty minutes and then to half an hour. It was just little by little, putting the right people in place to move in the direction we wanted to go. Our team had to be willing to accept things were going to change and do the things we needed to do to get to the next level.

Our doctors are not directly involved in management. It's really not what they're skilled at. They are strictly involved in providing patient care. The most productive use of a doctor's time is seeing patients."

Scan this QR code to learn more about Dr. Fishbein's case study.

You may have a completely different vision for your practice. If you set a goal, create a plan, and track the metrics that show where you are with your goal, you will get there if you do what it takes. Ultimately, the formula for growing an orthodontic practice and making your vision a reality only involves four principles:

1. The orthodontist is a technician, not a manager (so hire a good one).
2. Training your team to follow the steps to convert every viable lead into a new patient (and there are no bad leads).
3. Marketing to attract the right leads.
4. Software that tracks your metrics and holds your team accountable for the goals you've set.

We've seen it work over and over again. Mastering these four principles will help you grow, whether you're a brand new practice or finding yourself stuck at a plateau fifteen years in.

Dr. Kristen Knecht opened the doors to her brand new practice just days before the COVID-19 pandemic hit. She knew Knecht Orthodontics needed a strong brand identity and an enjoyable experience that would convert potential leads into happy patients in her practice from the very beginning. We ensured that her vision for her practice was reflected in her digital platforms using HIP's Brand Identity Process. In addition, Dr. Knecht onboarded the right team members who could truly be brand ambassadors. We then ensured every team member was well versed in our Patient Acquisition and Retention Framework™. Once we were confident they could convert the leads we generated, we launched her marketing campaigns.

Because Dr. Knecht followed the four principles for growing an orthodontic practice, we could track her results using software to follow up on metrics and keep her team accountable. In the first ten months after opening her doors during a pandemic, she converted over half a million dollars worth of digital leads into happy patients.

> *"I know doctors who work five or ten years to get to this level, and it's all happened so quickly. I couldn't have done that on my own."*

She produced well over a million dollars in her first full year in practice (2021).

Scan this QR code to learn more about Dr. Knecht's case study.

Most practices think that all they need is lead generation when they start working with us. "I just need more new patients!"

is what I frequently hear. The truth is, they don't just need lead generation. They need a team that can use the tools and the processes we provide to deliver an excellent patient experience. Otherwise, they have a massive leaky bucket and squander tons of opportunities without knowing what's happening. This concept is so important that I decided to dedicate a whole book to the critical role of your front desk and scheduling coordinators and how it can significantly impact the success of your practice.

Dr. Jennifer Eisenhuth had been in practice for around fifteen years when she realized she was stuck and needed a boost. She had been doing her own local marketing and just wasn't getting the desired results. She tried out a couple of marketing companies and found them helpful, but the results came in little steps here and there.

I liken HIP to being a rocket ship. It was amazing. What was exciting about working with HIP on a long-term basis was that they continued to grow with me and got better at what they were doing. And so we grew together.

Scan this QR code to learn more about Dr. Jennifer's case study.

The key to this kind of growth with marketing is having all four growth principles in place when you start running the campaigns. That's why we partner with the practices that we work with. We don't want to get lumped in with all the marketing guys that just redo your website, tweak your SEO, and run ads. All those vanity metrics like clicks and impressions tell you nothing. We measure the success of our partners through return on investment (ROI) by dividing the dollars brought in from starts due to marketing over the amount invested in the practice growth system. The numbers we get are staggering.

For example, we ran an ROI calculation on one of our partners, All Smiles Orthodontics, at their 14-month mark. In May 2020, they invested $171,500.00 into their practice. By August 2021, their amount returned ended up being just over $1,000,000.00. That's an $828,500.00 investment gain and an ROI of 483.09%! And that was only from patients who had started treatment. We didn't even show you the potential they could make from the production of leads in the pipeline. We'll get to that later.

We've talked about training your team to capitalize on the leads generated through marketing. Still, the big thing that we found was that 99.9% of orthodontic practices did not use Customer Relationship Management (CRM) software to follow up with prospective patients. They have their practice management suite that creates a file on a new patient when they are scheduled, but what about the leads coming in through the marketing efforts? These names and numbers are often scribbled down on sticky notes with a mental note to call them when I have a moment. In this day and age, there are so many distractions, so we end up not doing what we say we will or remembering to do it later. We see this all the time when we secret shop a practice. Nine out of ten times, we never got a callback, which is ridiculous! Returning that phone call is MONEY (and you help more people get the smile they want)! You'll learn more about our Secret Shop Report Card in Chapter 7 and if you would like to get a secret shop done on your front desk free of charge, simply scan this QR code to complete the form on our web page.

CRM software is very powerful, but it is also complicated. Our goal at HIP was to find out where all the leads that our marketing had generated went. Because no one used CRM for tracking, the leads all ended up going into the big void, and we could not tell if any of our efforts were affecting the practice growth and hitting the orthodontist's goals. We just wanted something that the scheduling coordinators could quickly and efficiently use to track the follow-ups on leads coming in and whether they converted to a new patient. That's why we built PracticeBeacon for orthodontic practices. You can discover more about its capabilities in Chapter 8.

Dr. Ernie McDowell, the founder of All Smiles Orthodontics, has five locations, so he definitely has a handle on the business perspective of orthodontics. When we partnered with All Smiles, Dr. McDowell wanted to leverage the power of modern marketing to grow his multi-location practice by converting more leads into patients. He wanted to invest more effort in lead follow-through with metrics that could be monitored and tracked. We trained his team to use our Patient Acquisition and Retention Framework™ so they were ready to handle the leads our marketing generated. We designed a fully-functioning website with effective search engine optimization (SEO) and implemented digital ad campaigns, retargeting ads, reputation management, and monthly email newsletters. To track the conversion of leads to new patients, we implemented the use of PracticeBeacon with his scheduling coordinators.

Applying the four principles of orthodontic practice growth gave All Smiles a five-times return on investment. Here's what Dr. McDowell had to say:

> *"You can learn and read about things that you need to do, but they don't teach you the follow-through and metrics you need to set up to provide checks and balances so you can track and monitor whether what you're doing is actually working. HIP actually sets that up for you, and they help you do it so you can really see that your investment is paying off. It makes you want to invest more because you know the value and the benefit. Marketing is an investment, and if you're doing it right, the more you market, the busier you should get. Eventually, your own rate-limiting factor should be your facilities and how much you want to work."*

It's important to note that Dr. McDowell is experiencing very rapid growth not only because he partnered with us, but because he only plays the doctor role and has a COO to run the day-to-day. You simply cannot do both if you want to grow.

Scan this QR code to learn more about All Smile's case study.

Despite the fact that the practices I have told you about are all very different, they all have a stellar front desk team or a patient care center, which you'll learn more about in Chapter 9. They invested in hiring the right people for the scheduling coordinator position and trained them to provide a WOW experience from the first call through every step of treatment. Most of all, they know that being an industry leader is a work in progress. They need to be able to rely on their team because they can't do it all.

You'll read about the "Ten Components for the Front Desk of Your Dreams" in the following chapters. These components are:

Chapter 1: A Team That Loves to Serve People
Chapter 2: A Team That Believes in Teamwork
Chapter 3: A Team That Exudes Positivity
Chapter 4: A Team That Understands Processes and Procedures
Chapter 5: A Team That Uses Simple Influence-Driven Scripts

Chapter 6: A Team That Embodies 'Speed to Lead'

Chapter 7: A Team That is Accountable

Chapter 8: A Team That Succeeds With Tracking and Transparency

Chapter 9: A Team That Benefits From a Patient Care Center

Chapter 10: A Team That Understands the Best Practices for Growth

Throughout this book, you will find case scenarios from Smith Orthodontics and their star scheduling coordinators: Jan, Lori, and Kim. This is a fictional practice that I created to illustrate key concepts that we encounter in real orthodontic practices daily. They have been doing things right, and they are seeing enormous growth. The other practices, team members, and results shared in this book are real examples of transformations we have seen firsthand. It is my hope that these examples, both made up and real, will help you to visualize a path to the creation of the front desk of your dreams.

CHAPTER 1

A Team That Loves to Serve People

I've had the opportunity to interact with team members from hundreds of orthodontic practices, both in person and by phone. Through thousands of touchpoints, whether observing an office visit, doing a secret shop, or listening to calls between scheduling coordinators and leads, I've noticed that the busiest practices all had one thing in common: the interaction with their team was enjoyable. Countless hours of analyzing great exchanges, horrible phone calls, and everything in between, have shown me one attribute that your front desk and scheduling team need: they must be a team that loves to serve people.

Let's bring this home. I want you to consider your front desk seriously. When you think about all the people you have interacting with leads and new patients in their first contact with your practice, is each committed to making the patient experience something memorable? Do they really love people? Can you hear the caring in their voice? Do people know they're in the right place before your team even opens their mouths? If your answers to these questions are yes, then congratulations! You've done a great job hiring, and we have the right people in place to build the front desk of your dreams. If not, you'll want to ask them whether they would like to step up or step out.

In far too many cases, when I talk to orthodontists and their office managers, the roles of the front desk and scheduling coordinator are overlooked and neglected: "It's a minimum wage job that nobody wants. How can we expect applicants to WOW us?" "It's only for the front desk... how amazing do they need to be?" Unfortunately, this thinking results in missed phone calls, gaps in your treatment coordinator's schedule, and lost income. The dollars you may have invested into marketing are generating leads that are now starting at another practice. Is this something you want? Excellent service is sadly a lost art.

When it comes to customer service, some companies have it nailed. Take Starbucks, for instance. They've taken their employees out of the mundane service industry by positioning them as baristas, completely changing their perspective of themselves. No matter what's going on in their lives, they assume the barista role and the standards that go with it when they come to work. They are there to serve and WOW people as they grab their coffee by brightening their experience. If you've ever received impeccable service from a barista at Starbucks, understand that dozens of hours went into training, coaching, and mentoring that individual to consistently maintain the standards that you and every customer has come to expect. Orthodontists need to learn from Starbucks about elevating the roles of the front desk and scheduling coordinators to a position that someone can enjoy and take pride in.

The culture at Starbucks was not established by accident. They had a straightforward goal: to create a culture that inspires others through excellence: in their products, people, and service. This simple goal took them from a small coffee shop in Seattle to a worldwide sensation (and a billion-dollar company). There are vast differences between a coffee shop and an orthodontic practice; however, the notion of employees providing excellent service to customers should remain consistent in every industry. If you visit different Starbucks stores around the globe, you will notice that while the food and beverages may be different, the standards and service provided are always consistent.

If you have been struggling to grow your practice, the first thing you need to do is cultivate a team that loves to serve people. Practices that make this their primary focus will have employees who value their work and their patients, strive to deliver exceptional service, and are eager to help grow your business.

Why do employees leave?

Unfortunately, in many practices and businesses, front desk customer service positions pay minimum wage, offer no benefits or perks, and are dead-end positions that provide minimal to no growth opportunities. Some scheduling coordinators also do records, work in the clinic, and more. So, they are doing numerous jobs for little pay and can't master one area of the practice. These types of jobs often have a high turnover rate, which affects the day-to-day life of the office and the overall morale of the workplace environment. To keep good team members and prevent high turnover, you need to make sure your practice is a great place to come to work. That includes:

- A fun, inviting culture.
- Key performance indicators for positions (so people can know if they are winning in the role).
- Proper training.
- Someone inspecting the metrics according to the goals and coaching when necessary (a lead or manager over the scheduling team).
- Incentives when goals are hit.
- Growth opportunities.

Most employees want a position where they can learn, grow, and contribute. Without these elements, your front desk and scheduling team won't feel inspired to do their jobs well, and they certainly won't feel motivated if they receive less than they deserve.

Let's think of Starbucks again. Yes, their baristas do start at minimum wage. Still, both full-time and part-time employees are entitled to health benefits, stock options, opportunities for career advancement (whether in retail or at the corporate level), vacation time, sick leave, and other great incentives. Also, team-building exercises, coffee tastings, team outings are regular events that contribute to the warm and upbeat Starbucks culture. Maybe you can't come anywhere close to that, but you don't have to pay a fortune to keep your team happy. You just need to install incentives and growth in the role and provide people with additional perks and rewards to help them love their jobs!

Make a goal, roll it out, and create a bonus pool. A good starting point could be the total number of new patients scheduled. For example, if the scheduling team hits the goal, 75 new patient consults are scheduled, and you know your treatment coordinator's average close rate is 70%, you will most likely start around 52 new patients. Would you pay your scheduling team $1,000.00 (shared evenly across the team) to hit your goal for the month? Simple incentives like this drive your team to move towards your desired outcomes.

What you DON'T want

If you've seen *Monsters Inc.,* you undoubtedly remember Roz, the scary old (monster) lady working at the front desk. With her raspy, monotone drawl, Roz delivers information in a manner that fits the stereotype perfectly: all people working in these roles hate their jobs and ultimately hate their lives. Roz is mean and lazy, and while she's entertaining to watch in an animated movie, the real-life version in an orthodontic setting would not be something to rave about. She is the perfect example of someone you DON'T want working at the front desk. If you don't know what I'm talking about, do a quick YouTube search and watch a video of Roz in action so you can understand what I mean. The bottom line is this: if you don't like people, this isn't the job for you. If you don't like talking to people, it's time to look for another job.

What you DO want

You DO want someone like Beverly, the Lead Front Desk Coordinator at Cassinelli, Shanker, and Baker Orthodontics. Beverly knows exactly what great service looks like, and she makes sure every patient, whether old or new, gets the same top-notch service:

> *"This lead came in from Facebook late last night. I saw it when I got into the office first thing in the morning, so I gave her a call. When the lady picked up the phone, I*

could hear it in her voice that I had awoken her from her sleep in her voice. I kind of panicked cause I didn't want her to get upset, so I introduced myself and apologized for interrupting her sleep. I told her I was calling her back to see if she'd want to schedule a new patient consultation at our office. I asked her if this was a good time to talk, and she said it was a good time to talk because I'd never catch her if she was awake!

We had a good laugh together. I went over everything and got all of her information. I tried to get her in that same day for her consult, but she told me she was super busy and couldn't leave work. Since we offer virtual consults, I told her it wasn't a problem if she couldn't get here. She loved that. I got her scheduled later that day. It made my morning, and she said it made hers, too."

There should always be a standard for your team to be pleasant, personable, and professional with patients. Outstanding service should occur when the initial phone call is made to a new lead, when they arrive for their consultation, and when they have future appointments. Providing outstanding service is ultimately how your practice will grow and how you can get to where you want it to be. If this is not currently happening in your practice, how will you fix it? It is important to visualize what you want the patient experience to look like and evaluate the steps you need to take to realize that vision.

Hiring The Right Candidate

It takes a lot of effort to go from where you currently are to where you want to be. You may not be hiring the proper people to fill these service roles or not coaching your team enough to maintain that quality service. Hiring a deadweight will only bring the rest of your team down. It can create a hostile work environment and leave patients with bad experiences in your practice. So, it would be wise to hire people who can provide the quality service you expect. Some questions you should ask yourself when interviewing candidates are:

- Do they often smile and make direct eye contact?
- Are they friendly, bubbly, and social?
- Do they exude confidence and professionalism?
- Do they have experience working in other customer service roles? How long did they last in these roles?
- Would this person get along well with the rest of my team?
- Are they willing to go above and beyond for patients?

If they're anything like Beverly, they should be someone you consider hiring. And if they're like Roz, run and steer clear!

Patient Care Position

If having a team that loves to serve people is the most critical component to achieving the front desk of your dreams, what is one quality each team member must have in common? Well, it's probably obvious by now, but they really should like being around people. And not just in a, *I'm nice to people at work because I have to be,* kind of way. It has to be genuine. They must love being around people and making them feel cared for. You must acknowledge that the people you hire for your front desk and scheduling team are in a "patient care" position, even though they do not provide health care services.

Your front desk and scheduling team are the mouthpieces between the practice, the doctor, and the patient. How they portray themselves to patients–their behavior, attitude, and demeanor–says a lot about you and your practice in general. It showcases the kind of people you hire and how you run your entire business. If you're in this position, you should care about your job, and if you don't, you should probably find something else to do. Patients aren't always going to be nice, but you still have to treat them with respect and empathy.

Sunrise Orthodontics receives great patient feedback daily, but it doesn't come easy. Some practices have this down perfectly, and it shows in their reviews. Julie, a Location Manager and Front Office Training Specialist at Sunrise, understands the importance of good service. If you do it right, it will reflect in your reviews. She takes pride in sharing this with new patients as she schedules their complimentary consultations:

> *"We have to work really hard for those reviews. If you go through all of them, you'll see five stars across the page,*

and almost all of them will say how great the team is or how much they love coming to our location because the people are so kind and helpful. So even though the doctors are doing a great job, people are commenting on how great the front desk team is. So I think that says a lot about the value of great service and how it can impact the overall patient experience. And so that says a lot about the kind of people you hire and how they provide patient care."

Adversity in the Workplace

Have you ever paid attention to how your front desk and scheduling team react during adversity? It is easy for people to provide quality service when the individuals they interact with are friendly and pleasant, but how do your employees respond to unfriendly and demanding patients? Are they still able to provide that same quality care? Every business has patients who are more challenging to deal with. In these situations, your front desk and scheduling team need to be as accommodating and respectful as possible, so your practice does not risk losing its business or jeopardizing its reputation.

That's why I think it's great for teams to engage in role-playing exercises to get used to what to say to patients when these difficult situations happen. And they do happen! For the patient role, just think of your favorite mean and grouchy TV character and pretend to be them, and for the scheduling coordinator role, think of the bubbliest person you know. It will help them address any future issues and doubles as a team-building exercise!

Investing in Your Employees

The best investment you can make for your practice is to apply the time, effort, and focus on service, as it can take your business from adequate to thriving. When you do this, your front desk will eventually grow your business and its reputation for you. Generally, a happy front desk and scheduling team will create satisfied patients who are willing to refer your practice to people they know and people they don't know (think Facebook, Twitter, Yelp, or Google reviews!). There are already so many practices doing this. For example, Dr. Connor Despot from Buda Orthodontics has a bonus structure for his front desk and scheduling team, where they get a $300.00 bonus if they decrease their missed call percentage by 2% over the last month. If you show your team that you appreciate their efforts and work ethic by investing in them, they will work harder to satisfy and exceed patient expectations and ultimately do their job better.

Manage Your Expectations

Your practice will not change dramatically overnight, and neither will your employees. Beverly understands the importance of being patient with your new hires as it will take time for them to get used to their new role and the standards:

> *"I always tell people that it will take at least six months before they feel entirely comfortable in this role. They*

know they have to provide quality service to patients, but there are also so many new tasks they will have to learn. I always tell my more experienced team to take the new hires under their wing. They have to see what it looks like and how to do it themselves. Shadowing them definitely helps them learn since you can only tell someone the facts so many times."

It is your job to make sure your new employees understand that it will take time to learn the nuances of the role and the standards and protocols of the practice. Make sure you let them know that there are no wrong questions and do what you can to make them feel comfortable along the way!

If you want to have this kind of team in your practice, the scheduling coordinator role needs to become a career that somebody wants to grow in. You may find yourself faced with the tough decision to let go of someone who has been with you for a long time. Trust me, in doing this, you are setting them free to be happier in their lives. You will make your whole team happier, and the quality of service will go up. Getting the right people in place is the first and most significant step you must take to grow your practice. The next thing to consider is the team dynamic: how well do they cooperate and work together to create the best outcome for everyone? That's why the next component of the front desk of your dreams is "A team that believes in teamwork."

CHAPTER 2

A Team That Believes in Teamwork

In a thriving orthodontic practice, every team member knows their role. How well they collaborate with the rest of your team impacts the performance of every position in your practice. For this book, we are simply focusing on the front desk and scheduling coordinator roles because of their critical importance to marketing and capitalizing on the generated leads. Most importantly, your bottom line is where you'll see the "teamwork making the dream work!" A culture that encourages asking questions and emphasizes coaching and mentoring will foster the growth and development you want.

What does a team player look like?

When my team at HIP and I start working with a new

practice, we always like to establish this one rule: "No onboard terrorists." I know this sounds a bit harsh, but I'm sure you've experienced how badly a person with a negative attitude can damage the morale and productivity of a whole team. Do you have someone who has toxic qualities? Maybe they're selfish, gossip or backstab others, or have a huge ego. That's an onboard terrorist, and we want to neutralize them quickly. It's far too costly to keep them. Instead, we like to hire people who have the qualities of a team player. Over the years, Julie has watched her team evolve into true team players:

> *"Someone who is a team player will actively work towards a solution. So even if it's not the solution they necessarily want, if it is what's best for the practice, they will work towards that together with the team. They're willing to take criticism and sacrifice their own comforts in the workplace just to have unity and work together like a well-oiled machine. My team has gotten a lot better at that. I feel like they all have strong team player attributes."*

In addition to this, there is also a need for team members to communicate effectively, manage conflicts, and lead collectively. Let's dig deeper into why these attributes make successful team players.

Effective Communication

Effective communication is essential to getting a new patient scheduled, whether in person or via phone, email, or text message. Your front desk and scheduling team must communicate well to do their jobs successfully and maintain a supportive environment.

According to Julie:

> *"Communication is one of the hardest things to master, but it's essential to work actively to improve it. It will make everyone's lives easier if we just learn to communicate better. You have to be super thorough in this job, and you have to express whatever you do effectively to the rest of your team. If you're working with a lead and need support from another team member, you have to relay the information to them as best you can so they have the whole story. They need to know as much as you know. If my scheduling coordinator needs to transfer a call to me, I want to know 'who, what, where, when, why, and how' before they do so to help the patient. Teamwork is meeting each other in the middle but allowing others to step in when support is needed. Communication helps make that process a lot more seamless."*

Conflict Management

Adversity is almost guaranteed in any workplace since we will not always see eye-to-eye with the people we work with daily. In group dynamics, it can be easy to get swept into drama and become involved in the conflicts of others. Addressing the matters directly and professionally will help avoid "going up the conflict escalator." Your team members should work towards de-escalating conflict, which can occur when each member actively listens to concerns, tries to understand perspectives, and works to uncover the root of the issues at play, which goes back to the need for effective communication.

On conflict, Julie shares:

> *"We really don't have many conflicts in our office because everyone has an amazing working relationship and they have great personalities. But when things get hectic, and the phone lines are ringing, and it gets hard to manage, sometimes it's easy to get irritated or annoyed with each other. It's just human nature. I make sure everyone has a role to play throughout the day so no one is confused about what they're doing. When everyone has a specialized role, we can control the hectic times better, and everyone can breathe a little easier. It goes back to communicating those roles effectively to avoid misunderstandings. Misunderstandings usually lead to conflict, so we want to avoid that."*

Collective Leadership

While there is usually one person in charge to manage and oversee the roles and responsibilities of team members, all team members need to approach the group dynamic with a collective leadership attitude. Doing so can generate higher quality engagement and investment within the team and let everyone take on a leadership role, regardless of their position. When you have team members who are using these skills effectively and consistently, they will strengthen the team dynamic and the overall success of your practice.

Julie encourages everyone to lead:

> *"I'm an office manager and trainer, but I spend a lot of the day supporting the front desk. I delegate the roles and tasks to the team and expect them to be on top of each of their duties since I want them to feel confident. This is especially important when a new hire needs to shadow experienced team members. That ability to own your role and teach it to others is so important because it shows they are confident to lead by example."*

Collaboration in the Workplace

Improving collaboration in your practice is not a daunting task: you really just need to encourage it to happen. Your employees may not even be aware that they can collaborate, so it is critical to let them know that helping each other is encouraged. Your practice will reach its goals and targets faster, overall morale in the workplace will improve, and the quality of work they produce will go up.

Creating a positive and supportive environment is essential for teamwork to flourish. Team members should feel like they are in a safe and welcoming environment. They should feel comfortable sharing their ideas, be encouraged to offer solutions to day-to-day problems and tasks, and receive praise for their contributions.

Things are happening at the front desk of a busy practice at lightning speed. Patients are coming and going, and the phone is usually ringing off the hook.

Let's think about this scenario: Jan and Lori are both scheduling coordinators at Smith Orthodontics. They are both following up with the leads that came in a few days prior. Jan calls one of the leads, Bill, and he answers quite annoyed: "I just received a call from you guys five minutes ago, and I told you I can't talk right now! I'm in a meeting! I will call you when I am free" and hangs up abruptly. Okay, Bill's not having the best day, but he didn't have to be so rude. Why wasn't Jan aware that Lori had already called him? Good communication avoids these kinds of situations.

With a proper system for follow-up and communication, Jan and Lori can avoid uncomfortable situations and WOW Bill with a few "love touches." This takes organization, notes on where the lead is in the pipeline, and communication. While I always encourage scheduling coordinators to follow a lead through to scheduling their exam, there are times when Jan and Lori will need to interact with each other's leads. If they can find out when the lead was last contacted and what was said, Jan can step in for Lori when Bill calls back and say something like, "Bill! We've been expecting your call. Lori told me you were in an important meeting. I hope it all went well. Let's see when we can get you in this week." Bill is now amazed that Lori took the time to tell Jan about him and that she cares enough to acknowledge how busy he is.

Using a customer relationship management (CRM) system is the best way to stay on top of leads. Otherwise, the leads can be tracked on paper or in a spreadsheet. However, these methods are not nearly as efficient. Our CRM software PracticeBeacon, which you will learn more about in Chapter 8, is designed specifically for orthodontic practices, is simple to use, and can help them do that quite effectively. Whatever method they use, communication is critical for successful collaboration between scheduling coordinators.

Set your team up for success!

When everyone has a defined role and is well trained in their skills, teams work better together. In many practices I visit, we see a front desk person who is the scheduling coordinator, the greeter, the treatment coordinator, and the list goes on. Sometimes when this person gets too busy, another front desk person is hired to help them, but now they have to train the new person on top of the job they have to do. I have never seen this work out well. For this reason, we often insist that practices hire people to fill specific roles before we even start working with them. In Chapter 10, you will see the organizational charts from the different busy and successful practices we support. Setting a practice up with roles other than the front desk and scheduling coordinator is the subject of Book 3 of the Orthodontic Practice Growth Series.

In most practices, the front desk performs the roles of answering the phones, greeting and scheduling patients, and coordinating the flow of the office. Chapter

9 discusses the advanced strategy of separating the role of interacting with leads for the first time from greeting them when they make their first visit to the office. This is a level of organization found in the busiest practices that we work with. Regardless of the strategy used in your practice, a clear definition of each team member's role is critical to a successful team.

Coaching and Mentoring

The most successful practices that I have come across have a culture where coaching and mentoring are encouraged between team members. The front desk and scheduling coordinator roles have a steep learning curve that requires guidance from the rest of the team. In many practices, we often find one superstar among a group of mediocre players. In the best practices, these superstars are recognized and encouraged to coach and mentor the rest of their team, giving them a hand up and elevating the whole team.

It is always such a pleasure to train with teams that embrace coaching and mentoring because there is a willingness to observe oneself grow. When this is part of the culture, giving and receiving feedback is a practiced skill, and people learn how to take it as a learning opportunity rather than a criticism of their shortcomings. Teams like this look forward to practicing new scripts and procedures by role-playing and helping each other become proficient in the interactions before they go live with patients. You can find tips on role-playing scripts in Chapter 5.

To effectively coach your front desk team members, you must first set clear goals, so they know what is expected of them and how they can accomplish the goals. If these goals are not being met, you must frame your feedback positively and respectfully.

I like the strategy for giving feedback that I learned from reading "The One Minute Manager" by Ken Blanchard and Spencer Johnson. It was first published in 1982, but the principles still have traction today. They have since published seventeen books related to this topic. The strategy goes like this:

1. Set three goals for each employee, which you can review in one minute or less.
2. Use a one-minute praise to give your employees positive feedback
3. Use a one-minute reprimand to express your dissatisfaction.

Julie from Sunrise uses this strategy often without even knowing it:

> *"One effective strategy is to lead with a compliment and provide feedback for improvement. So if I'm listening to one of my new trainee's calls and I hear them speaking with a patient, and they don't have that bubbly tone I'm looking for, I'll pull them aside afterward to coach them.*

I'll first give a compliment like, "I like how informative you were when you explained that to the patient."Then, I'll follow up with something I'd like them to improve by saying, "Next time, try using a friendlier tone as it will help the patient feel more comfortable." I'll pay attention to that again when I hear them on the next phone call to make sure they are implementing my feedback."

The next component of the front desk of your dreams is like the systems check you need to make sure your team is firing on all cylinders and ready for flight. Attitude is everything, so you need a team that exudes positivity. Once we have a team that believes in teamwork, we're just about ready to add the rocket fuel and take off.

CHAPTER 3

A Team That Exudes Positivity

When you put together a team of great people who love to serve, we can usually assume that they have positive attitudes, but it is not something that can be left to chance. When you take the time to think about it, we are expecting people to take time out of their busy lives, come into our practice, commit to a treatment plan that takes a long time, is uncomfortable, and requires discipline, and we want them to pay a lot of money to do this! We better keep them focused on the positive aspects of care, like the beautiful smile we build together. We have to ooze positivity, enthusiasm, and excitement about the long game so they stay focused on the goal. That's why I decided to dedicate a whole chapter to positivity.

Your front desk and scheduling team must be willing to go above and beyond for patients and be excited to work together to achieve shared goals. It is inspiring when you have finally found the individuals who can make this happen. Unfortunately, one bad attitude has the potential to corrupt everything you have worked so hard to achieve. Think back to a time when you encountered someone with a negative attitude. Perhaps they complained constantly: about the weather, their friends, their job, and even their family members. Maybe they were always spreading rumors or gossiping about others: "Did you hear Jane did this?... Fred told me not to say anything, but this happened." Or it may be that they were just unpleasant to be around and never had anything nice to say. After being in the presence of this person over an extended period, you most likely felt emotionally drained and desperate to leave their vicinity. We have all been there. I sure have.

You don't want this kind of person working in your practice. Their "onboard terrorist" qualities that we introduced earlier can create a toxic work environment for everyone involved. So, how can you cultivate a team that exudes positivity? This chapter will determine the consequences of negative thinking in the workplace and the benefits of developing a team that is overflowing with happiness and joy to grow your practice in a meaningful way.

Negative Thinking in the Workplace

Negative thinking can severely impact your front desk team dynamic and overall workplace morale. Thoughts connect to other thoughts and create a downward spiral. Once you think of one bad thing, it polarizes you, and your emotional disposition starts to shift. You start frowning, the corners of your mouth turn down, and your tone of voice changes. This disposition rubs off on other team members but more importantly, it affects the leads and patients. People start questioning whether they want to be around you or not. Your teammates start to avoid you, and appointments start to cancel. It's almost like you put new patient repellant on! We just can't have this! A bad attitude costs you money.

Catch It Early!

Catching these behaviors and attitudes should happen as early as the interview process. An excellent way to determine if your potential candidates have these negative qualities is by asking the right questions and paying attention to what they say and how they say it. Additionally, paying attention to their tone and body language can help you determine if they would be a good fit for your practice. Ask yourself: Would this person get along with the rest of my team? Do they seem like they can be a team player? Are they willing to go above and beyond for patients? Are they exuding positive energy that my team and I would benefit from being around? Suppose you notice that a potential candidate focuses on their strengths, desires to improve their weaknesses, and demonstrates their willingness to grow within a collaborative setting. You probably want this person on your team.

Alyx, the Director of Patient Communications at Fishbein Orthodontics, knows what to look for when hiring a new employee:

> *"Hiring for personality is number one. You can teach anyone a skill, but you can't teach personality. We're looking for somebody who, in the interview, asks questions, smiles and laughs with us, and shares great stories and examples. If they're shut off, cold, or just not engaged in the process, we automatically know they're not who we're looking for."*

We have to acknowledge that we are all human, and we can't all be beacons of positivity at every moment of the day. We all have good and bad days. However, there is a difference between being in a bad mood and having a negative attitude: a bad mood is temporary, while a negative attitude is a state of mind. If the case arises where a previously positive employee begins to develop a poor attitude, it is essential to determine the root cause of that behavior. Try speaking with that employee directly and offering your support–perhaps they need sympathy and active listening to work out an issue in their personal life or have had difficulty dealing with a specific patient. Whatever it may be, taking the appropriate corrective measures to address the issue directly will ensure they understand that a level of positivity and professionalism is expected from them to fulfill the needs of the patients and the practice.

Alyx believes:

> *"You need to have a team that is excited and onboard to service your patients. Coming to work with a positive attitude every day is what's going to set your team apart. If someone is having a bad day and projecting that onto your patients, they're going to feel it; it can turn a great phone call into a sour one, really quick. That's not the goal. We want our patients to call us when they are having a bad day and for us to turn it around. If you have negative people, you're not going to be able to do that.*
>
> *I can read my team: I know them, I pay attention to them, so if somebody is having a bad day or they seem off, I always pull them aside and ask if they're okay. A lot of the time, something is going on at home or in their personal life. You have to be empathic in those moments and reach out by saying you're sorry they're feeling this way, and if they need to take a day off, that's fine. But ultimately, we are here to provide an experience to our patients, which we have to stick to."*

The consequences of negative thinking are too costly to bear. Whenever you can address it early, turn it around, and encourage your team members to practice achieving a positive state of mind. If you do not see changes, you should track and monitor their behaviors and take the disciplinary actions required to ensure your practice runs the way you have envisioned it. Share positive stories, tools, and strategies for getting into the zone of positivity to elevate the overall work environment.

Positive Thinking in the Workplace

Positive thinking can allow your team to overcome adversity more seamlessly, share information and ideas more effectively, and make more informed and thoughtful decisions. It can significantly impact workplace morale by increasing productivity, collaboration, and teamwork. A positive attitude can also be infectious and contagious. When positivity becomes the expected norm for your practice, you will be amazed by all the other extraordinary attributes it inspires. Your practice will become more efficient, and your team will show more initiative, solve problems more quickly, and go the extra mile to satisfy your patients. The result is improved customer service, lower turnover, and increased job satisfaction.

Much like everything else we have discussed, it begins with you, your vision, and how well it is conveyed to your team. The team leader must be the role model for this type of thinking and behavior. No matter what is going on in your life, it is crucial to show up to work every day with a smile on your face, your head held high, and your posture as straight as an arrow. Get your team pumped at the beginning of the day, celebrate successes and accomplishments frequently, and reward your team for a job well done. Discuss the vision and mission statement with the team during meetings, make reasonable and achievable goals and targets, and effectively coach and mentor your team when these objectives are not met. It begins with you, but it will transfer throughout your team. Before you know it, all your team members will be excited to come to work and eager to do their best daily.

Alyx knows the importance of leading by example:

> *"You have to lead by example. Look, we all have things going on in our lives, but you gotta come in and be excited. I try to get my team pumped up, ask them how they're all doing, offer coffee to everyone. I want to get their energy up so they can spread that to other people. You have to try to instill that attitude in your team; it's so important."*

A positive attitude is a driving factor that can turn a fixed mindset into a growth mindset. A person with a fixed mindset thinks they are who they are and cannot change. They see others as being endowed with skillsets that they did not get when they were handed out. They feel disadvantaged and unable to change. Fortunately, being immersed in a culture of positivity can help shift a person's mindset from fixed to growth. When your team focuses on improving their growth mindset, they are more likely to cultivate change through their own personal and collaborative efforts and less likely to see themselves as individuals who are incapable of doing so. People with growth mindsets see challenges as opportunities to learn and acquire new skills. They see failures as moments to learn from their mistakes and come back stronger than before. These are the types of people who should be working in your practice.

Julie understands how important it is to hire the right kind of people:

> *"I feel like the majority of people we hire are positive thinkers. They're going to take the time to sacrifice their time to create a solution for patients, parents, members of the team, and for the sake of the practice. They're going to get the job done because they maintain that kind of attitude. The people we've hired in the past that don't think that way have never worked out. They ended up leaving within the year we hired them."*

Once a practice gets these first three components handled, they have the foundation that we can work with for practice growth. We've got the right people with the right attitude to learn what they need to do to build the practice that you have envisioned. Do we start marketing yet? Not quite. We need to make sure that the precious leads we generate are taken care of properly so that they become our valued patients. For that to happen, read on to learn to discover the processes and procedures for training your team.

CHAPTER 4

A Team That Understands Processes and Procedures

If attitude were everything, everyone would be a superstar when starting a new job. If you hired the right people based on the previous chapters, these people show up with enthusiasm and eagerness to please. Sadly, when the front desk and scheduling coordinator role is considered just reception, people develop their ideas about the job. The front desk is primarily about getting the leads that contact your practice to schedule a consultation and then getting those consultations to show up to start treatment. If your front desk team cannot do this, it does not matter how many ads you place or how much marketing you do. The leads will fall through the cracks, and the money will be wasted.

It comes down to this: anybody that handles new patient phone calls and scheduling has the most critical role in the practice. The treatment coordinators can only do their jobs if they have exams scheduled for them, and that is the responsibility of the front desk: to schedule those opportunities and get them in the chair. They drive and dictate the volume of production more than anybody. So, how can you make sure your team does it efficiently? It all comes down to training your team on the proper processes and procedures. If you consistently show them what you are looking for and give them the tools to succeed, there's no reason why they won't be able to schedule hundreds of prospective patients to fill those chairs every month. However, to do this successfully, your team must understand the central aspect of their role: to be true sales professionals.

You should not take the front desk role lightly. The front desk and scheduling team are not supposed to be warm bodies with a pulse, doing mundane daily tasks. They should not be making people feel as bored and resentful as they do, whether on the phone or in person, solely because they hate their minimum wage job. What they should be doing every day is showing up with the right attitude and goal to make a sale. And to make sales, they have to show people why they believe in the products and services they are selling. How, you may ask, are they selling if they're not the ones making the deals and signing the contracts? Before we answer this question, it's essential to determine what sales is.

What it means to be in sales

The word 'sales' sometimes has a negative connotation associated with it. It is often perceived as someone trying to convince you to buy something you don't need or someone pushing you to close on something. It's an effort to try to get money out of you. However, everything is sales. The word sales itself means helping people! If you don't believe me, just look at the word's etymology. The infinitive 'to sell' comes from the old English word 'sellan,' which means 'to give.' Unfortunately, the definition became negative somewhere along the line (possibly due to Hollywood stereotypes of salespeople). But, to sell means to give. If you are operating out of integrity, you give people your time. In a new patient consult, you're giving people your time by providing them with information. But, you are also giving them wisdom, perspective, empathy, value, advice, and coaching.

How are they selling if they're not making the deals and signing the contracts?

The answer to this is simple: if you miss just one new patient call per day, that's one million dollars of revenue loss at the end of the year. Therefore, if your front desk and scheduling team is missing ten calls per day, that's $10,000,000.00 in revenue lost at the end of the year. On the other hand, if they schedule ten new patients per day, that's $10,000,000.00 in revenue gained at the end of the year if your treatment coordinator can get them started! Your front desk and scheduling team are the first individuals who can take your patients from where they currently are to where they want to be by selling them products and services that will get them there. Once your team is clear on where these leads want to be, selling comes into play. So, you need to instill in your team that 80% of growth and success is in their mindset and philosophy. They will do it if they believe they can sell it and have the tools to do it efficiently. The remaining 20% is the physical mechanics of actually making it happen!

The interested leads will take the time to go to your website, put in their information, and request an appointment. There's a reason why they did that, but they may not be fully committed. They are guarded against all the negative stereotypes associated with what they think sales is.

How can your front desk team lower the guards of prospective patients?

As sales professionals, it should be the goal and vision of your team members to establish that trust and connection to get people to let down their defenses.

There are numerous ways you can train your team to do this.

Show your true intentions:

You want to be influential, not persuasive. Persuasion is pushing somebody and convincing somebody to take something they don't need, isn't going to help them, and isn't a good decision. But it's a good decision for you because you get a commission check and bonus. Influence, on the other hand, is a good deed. Influencing someone to make the best decision comes from a place of integrity. If it's a good fit and a good decision for them, closing somebody is one of the best gifts you can give. If you can't close them, you can't help them. If you can't close the contract, you can't make their teeth look good. If it's the right fit, and you know that your product or service will help this person, it is your job to do your best to influence them to say yes.

Understanding that everybody is afraid and defensive helps us to approach them with empathy in this process and truly serve them. When you want nothing but the best for the person you're speaking to, that message gets transmitted, even through the phone. With this intention in mind, you can forget all about sleazy salespeople and help patients get the beautiful smiles they desire.

Use softer language:

A subtle shift in language can open up a whole new

window to how people perceive your words and receive what you're trying to tell them. The best words to use are softening words: possibly, maybe, convenient, and appropriate. Take a look at how these phrases are different:

- So, the next step would be to go ahead get a consultation scheduled so we can get you in to see [doctor's name].
- So, the next step would be to book an initial consultation... we actually have some openings tomorrow, if that might possibly be convenient for you?

The first sentence is presumptuous. You're assuming the patient is ready to schedule and come into the practice, and it might be a little persuasive. The second sentence, on the other hand, sounds softer. The ball is in the patient's court, but you are softening your tone to not sound too pushy.

Look at another example of setting the frame for the same-day start using softer language. This is what we call a "trial close," as we are pre-framing what will happen to set the right expectations for a same-day start:

- So, the way the appointment is going to go is: you're going to come in and you're going to meet [TC's name], the treatment coordinator. She's fantastic! We're going to take some photos and records, and the doctor is going to take a look at [patient's name]. If [doctor's name] does decide that [patient's name] is ready for treatment, we could get [patient's name] back into the clinic the same day so that you don't have to come back for another appointment, if that might be convenient for you?

Another way to help people lower their guard is to take big, scary concepts and make them make sense by using "kinda like" bridges. Here's an example:

- It's kinda like [insert DIY company], but you actually get to work with an actual doctor, and your teeth aren't going to fall out of your face (LOL).

Change your tempo and tonality:

When you're on the phone or in the consultation room, you can change the vibe of how words and language are received by saying the same thing in two different ways. So pay attention to the two T's, tonality and tempo, since they're the keys to the kingdom. You should always sound skeptically optimistic whenever you talk to a prospective patient. Keep your tone always upbeat but framed with a hint of doubt. Here's an example:

- I see that you took some time to request an appointment with us. Is that right?

Use connecting phrases:

It's all about impact versus information: you want to

make an impact, not just give information. Connecting phrases are how we take information and make it impactful. Some examples of connecting phrases are:

- In order to
- So that you
- Which means you
- Without having to
- Which will allow you to

Take a look at this example of how to use them:

- In order to save you time, we can actually start treatment that same day, which means you won't have to come back for another appointment! If that is possibly more convenient for you?

Using connecting phrases is most important in the trial close on the new patient call and at the end of the consultation when you're trying to make the same-day start.

Chunk down your spiel:

Don't reveal everything at once! People's guards are up, so they're deaf to whatever you're saying. If you chunk it up into three or four segments, it's softer, and they have a moment to digest the information. There's power in the pause. Get comfortable with the awkward pauses. Don't fill in the silence. Put your phone on mute if you need to. Soft, slow, pause; it's powerful.

Analyze these two examples:

Example 1:

- *Hello?*
- *Hi [patient's name], this is [your name] from [practice name]. I'm calling regarding a recent appointment you requested on Facebook for a consultation. I can provide you with information and set up an appointment if you'd like. Is this a good time to talk?*
- *Uh, sorry, where did you say you're calling from?*

Example 2:

- *Hello?*
- *Hello, is this [patient's name]?*
- *Yeah, may I ask who's calling?*
- *Hi, this is [your name]. I'm giving you a call from [practice name]. [Pause and give them a moment to digest and see if they recognize you].*
- *Oh, yes, hi, how are you?*
- *I'm good, how are you?*
- *Good thanks. I was giving you a call because you took some time to request a consultation with us. Is that right?*
- *Yes, I did.*
- *Great, is this a good time to talk?*

In the first example, the scheduling coordinator isn't allowing the patient to get a word in. She's revealing all the information at once from the beginning. In the second example, we break the information down and allow the patient to recall her request while finding out more about her. This also gets her talking a bit more, which will lower her guard.

Step-by-Step Procedures

Now that you understand what these calls should sound like, we will review the procedures.

How-To...

Answer the phone:

Get into the habit of letting people know you are there to help them. A great way to do this is by ditching the standard phrase "can I help you?" and replacing it with "I can help you!"

Saying this will show them you are eager to serve their needs and help them with all their inquiries. Look at how impactful it is in comparison to the standard response:

- *Hello, this is [your name]. How can I help you?*
- *Hello, this is [your name]. I can help you!*

If a prospective patient asks you about pricing over the phone, don't shut them down. If someone asks how much it'll cost, don't say, "We don't give any quotes over the phone," in a condescending tone. Always provide them with an answer, even if you are unsure what their treatment costs will look like. Pushing back and not explaining pricing is not a good idea. They will call somewhere else and get the answer they're looking for.

Similarly, don't drop the big number if they ask how much treatment costs. Prospective patients will be turned off if they hear from the beginning that the treatment will cost them $6,000.00. When you see car advertisements on TV, they don't lead by saying, "This Audi will cost you $50,000.00." Instead, they will give you a down payment percentage and the lowest monthly fee. It's essential to do the same when discussing average treatment costs. The strategy of not discussing fees is not going to help your practice. Instead, give prospective patients accurate, digestible numbers.

Here's what you can say if a prospective patient is asking you about fees in your initial conversation:

- *We have to see you to provide a treatment plan with accurate fees, but treatment typically starts at [insert your average downpayment and monthly payment] (ex. $300.00/down and $149.00/month). Would something like that work for you?*

Then, GO SILENT.

- *Great! When can you come in this week for your*

free consultation?

Place people on hold:

Sometimes, we get busy and inevitably have to put people on hold. Have you ever called a company to inquire about their services, and when they answered, they quickly responded with, "Hello, please hold." Then the annoying background music comes on, leaving you no opportunity to respond? Yeah, I'm sure we've all experienced that at some point. And let's be honest, it can be an instant turn-off. We might even end up hanging up without feeling bad about it. That is called a dry hold in business. You may be thinking, Well, my practice doesn't do that. We aren't THAT bad. But are they doing this?

- *Thank you for calling [practice name]. Can I place you on a quick hold?*

Yeah, that's a nicer dry hold. Better, but not great. And here's why. The prospective patient can hang up at any point during that hold, and if they do, you haven't collected any of their information. You have no idea who they are. And they probably won't call back. They'll call somewhere else, losing you a new lead and possible revenue. Instead, train your team on the wet hold. Here's what it looks like:

- *Thank you for calling [practice name]. This is [your name]. I can help you!*

- *Ok, great! I'm happy to help you with that. May I ask for your name and number in case we get disconnected?*

Then, log this information into your system!

- *Ok, [patient's name], I need to place you on a very brief hold while I do x, y, z. Is that ok?*
- *Great, I will be right back!*

Now, you know who they are, you have their information, AND it's in your system. If they have to hang up, you can always call them back.

How to respond when a patient says they will call you back:

Don't wait for the patient to call you back. Once a patient is off the phone, the odds of them calling you back soon is very slim–they will forget or won't consider it a priority. They may get back to you in a few weeks or even search for another orthodontic practice. Instead, ask them when a good time would be for you to call THEM back. You can say something like:

- *You can call me back, but we like to schedule call-backs just for your convenience. We want to make it simple and easy and provide you with a great experience. How's tomorrow at 1:00 pm, or Monday at 8:00 am?*

Use Google Calendar, Outlook, or PracticeBeacon, and

make a task to call that person back at that time.

How to edify the doctor/team/office on a scheduling call:

You want to sell the practice you work for to make a sale. It's that simple. You have to show patients why your practice is better than the competition. Let your prospective patient know why your practice is an excellent choice for them and their needs. Here's what you can say:

- *Let me tell you a bit of [practice name or doctor name] and what makes us different....... [short soundbite on the mission/values as well as a short blurb about the doctor[s]].*

Schedule a patient:

We live in a time in which consumers want everything NOW. When prospective patients call, fill out a form, or opt in via an ad, the best thing you can do to CONVERT that prospect into a patient is to schedule their new patient consult ASAP.

- *When would you like to come in tomorrow [or this week]?*

Let them know you have open spots for them, or you can fit them in at a time that works best for them. As Alyx says, *"Even if you're fully booked, make it happen."*

Respond when someone cannot come in within 72-hours:

We have busy lives, so we expect that people can't take time out of their schedule to attend an appointment right away. The beautiful thing about today's world is the access to the internet and video conferencing. It's made our lives that much easier, especially when the world shut down for two years because of a pandemic. Provide your prospective patients with the option of a virtual consult with a treatment coordinator. The patient can do it from the comfort of their own home and minimize the impact on their time and schedule. You'll learn more about virtual consults in Chapter 6.

Follow-up before an appointment to prevent no shows:

Send a text message or phone them the morning of their appointment. There's nothing worse than putting your effort into a conversation with someone who doesn't plan on showing up. Here's what you can say:

- *Hey [patient's name]! We are looking forward to seeing you at 1:00 pm today! If you need directions, here is a link to our listing [insert google maps link]. This should open on maps and bring you straight to us! Let me know if you have any questions. P.S. Ask for [your name] when you get here!*

What else should you know?

There may be other inquiries or questions you will need to know when speaking with prospective patients. The most frequently asked questions by patients usually relate to payment, insurance, and treatment. Therefore, it would be wise to provide your front desk and scheduling team with a list of frequently asked questions (FAQs) they may encounter outside of what is mentioned in this book. Scan this QR code to access a list of FAQs suggested by the American Association of Orthodontists that might be relevant to your particular style of practice.

This is an excellent opportunity to work collaboratively with your team to develop the correct responses that suit your business needs and requirements. That way, your team can have them readily accessible with short scripts to relay the answers to patients properly.

Once your front desk and scheduling team are trained to handle calls and schedule leads, it's time to turn on the marketing. You can spend the marketing dollars with confidence once you know that your team will care for those leads and nurture them into new patients in your practice.

Remember the four principles for growing an orthodontic practice from the introduction:

1. The orthodontist is a technician, not a manager [so hire a good one].
2. Training your team to follow the steps to convert every viable lead into a new patient [and there are no bad leads].
3. Marketing to attract the right leads.
4. Software that tracks your metrics and holds your team accountable for the goals you've set.

As the leads begin contacting your practice, read on to find out exactly what to say to them so that they schedule their free consultation and show up for that appointment. The next chapter on simple scripts provides the words and language that convert hundreds of leads into new patients every month for our busiest practices.

CHAPTER 5

A Team That Uses Simple Influence-Driven Scripts

While nobody wants to sound like a robot, saying exactly the same thing to everyone in a mechanical voice, it's also no fun to stammer and lose your words because you don't know how to handle a particular conversation. Simple scripts that pertain to specific discussions and situations that come up frequently can help team members to develop their proficiency in knowing exactly what to say every time. Of course, we want your personality to shine through, and we definitely need you to be natural and present with the person you are speaking to. Having a script provides a starting point with all the milestones we hit in a particular conversation.

Businesses usually use simple scripts to help teams stay on track and keep conversations focused and precise. You want to avoid calling the patient multiple times for different information, so scripts can help employees get all the information they need in one simple phone call. The scripts should provide the bare bones and not be lengthy and thorough. More in-depth conversations should be left for the in-person consultation. As policies in the practice change, the script should also change since they should always be up-to-date. And these scripts do not need to be followed precisely! You can take the script and make it your own to feel more natural to you, as long as you provide the essential information. This chapter will provide you with simple scripts to use for phone calls and text messages and some prompts for role-playing exercises to ensure your team is successfully integrating the scripts into their conversations with prospective patients.

What should your scripts look like?

It is essential to make sure your scripts are kept short and sweet. Ensure that you stay on topic and keep it brief to make this happen. The necessary information should be left for the consultation, and too many details over the phone can lead to confusion. Also, don't answer questions they don't ask. Your exchange should be smooth and productive if you stay close to the script. Before starting the phone call, keep in mind that you are trying to provide a convenient service to the patient. You want them to know you are there to minimize the impact of their time since you are aware of how busy the day can get. Also, remember that you can use a virtual consult to pre-qualify new patient opportunities. Make sure you suggest this to them once you have them on the phone ready to book or via a text or email.

Script 1: Pre-Qualifying New Patient Opportunities

Phone Call:

Ensure the patient is aware that the virtual consult will jumpstart treatment by allowing them to get their full treatment breakdown, answers to their questions, and an idea of how much everything will cost–without them having to leave their house! They will be able to schedule the in-practice visits more efficiently, helping them save time off from work or school.

Script Option 1

- *Hi [patient's name], you will love our virtual process! I will text/email you some easy instructions to begin. You simply answer a few questions, submit a few photos of your teeth, and we will be back in touch with all of the information you need to get started with your treatment, including fees!*

Script Option 2

- *Our first appointment is [next day available], but we can go ahead and get the process started today. We will text you some simple instructions, and all you have to do is answer a few questions and submit a few photos of your teeth. We will get back to you later today with a Free Quote, and then our Treatment Coordinator can call to review the quote and the next steps. How does that sound?*

Text Message:

Here's the follow-up text message you can send to the patient after you've prefaced everything over the phone:

- If texting the patient directly:
    - *Hi [patient's name], we're so excited to help you with your orthodontic needs. Here are the photos of your teeth we need to get started with your Free Quote. Once I get your photos, we will be in touch with the quote and treatment plan within an hour! P.S. I may have a few questions based on your photos!*
- If texting a parent:
    - *Hi [parent's name], [patient's name] is due for a follow-up visit with [doctor's name]. Can you text us these photo angles to evaluate treatment virtually and see if an in-person visit is needed? If everything looks good, then we can save you a trip!*

You can also use this for observation/recall and retainer patients!

Script 2: New Patient Flow

Your first conversation with a patient will impact them, so you should definitely pay attention to what you're saying and how you're saying it. Keep in mind everything we discussed in the previous chapter: your tone and tempo should be skeptically optimistic. You shouldn't reveal too much information at once (chunk it down) and answer prospective patients' questions to the best of your ability.

Greeting and Information Gathering:

- *Thank you for calling [practice name]. My name is [your name]. I can help you!*
- *Ok, great! I'm happy to help you with that. May I ask with whom I'm speaking?*
- *Thank you, [patient's name]. I'm happy to answer any questions. Would you mind giving me a good phone number to reach you if we get disconnected?*
- *Awesome! Do you have a few minutes right now for me to gather a little bit of information so that I can help you get scheduled??*
    - If yes, say:

-Ok, great, and proceed to set up a consultation appointment.

- If no, say:

  -Got it. Is there a timeframe for us to check back with you?

Patient Bonding Questions:

- *How did you hear about us? OR Who can we thank for referring you to us?*
- *How long h*ave you been considering coming to see us?
- *Do you have any main/specific concerns about [the treatment needed]?*
- *Will this appointment be for you or someone else?*
- *Was there anyone in the family considering treatment who might want to be seen?*

What Makes [Practice Name] a Great Choice:

- *Let me tell you a bit of [practice name] and what makes us different... [short soundbite on the mission and values as well as a short blurb about the doctor[s]].*

- Examples:
  - The doctor has been in practice X years
  - Board-certified, voted best practice, top 1%

Invisalign Provider

- Retainers For Life program
- The doctor is a native of the area
- Our mission is for top-quality care at an affordable cost for everyone
- Fun environment, play area for kids, snacks for all patients
- Multiple convenient locations, same-day braces, fast appointments
- In-network with most insurances to make it easy for you

Gathering Patient Information:

- Patient Name OR Name of the responsible party and who is bringing them
- Birthday
- Address
- Best phone number
- Alternate phone number
- Best email address
- Allergies or medical concerns
- Name of their general dentist
- Approximate date of last dental cleaning
- Any insurance you would like us to check for you?
    - Insurance company
    - Insurance ID #

Appointment Setting:

- *Ok, great! Thank you for all of that information. Did you have a date/time that works best for you to come in, or would you like me to give you our soonest availability?*
- *Do you prefer morning or afternoon?*
- *We have an X day at X time or a Y day and Y time. Does one of those work better for you?*

**If you offer a free consultation, explain that fully here, then make the ask for the actual appointment.

Price & Fee Question Handling:

- *We do need to see you for an exam, which is free of charge, to give you an accurate fee and treatment plan, only because the fee totally depends on how long the doctor says you will need to be in treatment. Some people are in treatment for 12 months, some for over 24 months.*
- *BUT what I CAN tell you is that we do have super affordable payment plans for everyone, all in house, at 0% interest to you, no credit checks, and most people are able to start treatment for as little as $X down and monthly payments as low as $X per month. Could that possibly work for you?*

Closing and Same-Day Start Trial Close:

- If an appointment is set:
  - *It was great speaking with you today [patient's name]. Did you have any other questions for us?*
  - *Ok, awesome! When you come in, you will meet with one of our awesome Treatment Coordinators, take some photos and x-rays together, and the doctor will do an exam. The consultation is free of charge to you. Please allow about one hour for your appointment. If the doctor does think that you're ready for treatment, we can actually go ahead and get your treatment started that same day so that you do not have to come back for another appointment, if that might be convenient for you?*
  - *Thank you so much for calling, and we look forward to seeing you at your appointment!*
- If no appointment is set:
  - *It was great speaking with you today [patient's name]. Thank you so much for calling, and we look forward to hearing from you again soon.*

Text Messages

We have also provided a curated list of text messages

you can send to patients to keep them informed along the way. Use them as building blocks, and feel free to customize them with your team members. For example, adding "happy [insert day of the week]! or hope you had a lovely weekend!" at the beginning of each message to provide a friendlier tone. It's convenient for your team as they will just need to do a quick copy, paste, and edit! Doing this will ensure your team isn't wasting time repeatedly sending the same message.

Same-day Appointment Confirmation Text:

- *Hey there, [patient's name]. It's [your name] at [practice name]! We are looking forward to seeing you today. Do you have our address, or would you like me to text it to you quickly so you can easily just click it when you get in the car?*

Post Phone Call + Voicemail - Connecting Text:

- *Hey there, [patient's name]. That was me who just called you! This is [your name] from [practice name]! I was just calling because I see that you requested a free consult for possibly looking at Braces or Invisalign treatment with [doctor's name]. Is that right? I just wanted to help you get that scheduled! Is there a day and time that works best for you to come in? Or when could be a good time to call you back to schedule? Looking forward to meeting you!*

Unresponsive After 48-72 Hours Text:

- *Hey there, [patient's name]. This is [your name] from [practice name]! How are you? I just wanted to chat quickly and see if you still might want to come in for a free consult for Braces or Invisalign treatment with [doctor's name]! Looking forward to hearing from you soon! :)*

More Messages in PracticeBeacon (the CRM we created)

With the click of a button, you can access more text responses that can be used to handle different booking scenarios. PracticeBeacon addresses the conversation immediately. You just have to navigate the conversation and choose the correct reply, and PracticeBeacon will send it out.

Scan this QR code to see more options you can use to facilitate timely and personable messages!

Role-Playing

During training sessions, get your team to role-play with one another! This is a great way to use simple scripts and practice them, so your team is ready to go when they do this live with patients. Set them up in pairs: one of them being the patient and the other the scheduling coordinator. Then, recast and reverse roles! You can do this in the form of a phone call, text message, or email. Use the scripts provided above to help guide your conversation.

Here are some role-playing prompts you can use with your team to help get them started:

- A lead just requested an appointment on Facebook 3 minutes ago.
- A prospective patient is in another country but would like to speak to someone for a consultation.
- A prospective patient has been scheduled for the following day, and you'd like to remind them about their appointment.
- A prospective patient left a voicemail on Friday morning and would like to be seen within 72 hours.
- A prospective patient only has time on Friday, but your TC is fully booked that day.
- A prospective patient you're speaking to cannot continue chatting due to an upcoming meeting.
- A prospective patient calls you, but you have a patient on the other line.

Remember!

Not every conversation with a prospective patient will go smoothly. If adversity arises during an interaction with a patient, there are a few things you should keep in mind when trying to get things back on track:

- Try to diffuse the situation as soon as possible and refrain from arguing with or interrupting the patient.
- Make sure you listen to all the patient's concerns and repeat them back to them to prove that you understand what they are asking.
- Respond to their concerns in a helpful, clear, and amenable tone. HOW you say things is typically more important than WHAT you say!
- Energy and excitement are everything!
- If the patient asks you a question that you don't know the answer to, put them on a wet hold. If the patient must be on hold for longer than two minutes, ask for their contact information and call them back so they aren't on hold for long periods.
- Ensure the patient understands you are trying to help them.

The TRUTH is that they took their time to reach out to you. You did not force them to call you. The FACTS are that there is a reason they took their time to do that!

Your mission is to serve them and build a bridge from where they are to where they want to be! The REALITY is that everyone is guarded. Remember that guarded does not mean not interested. Guarded just means guarded. You can lower their guard to create a connection with a fun, upbeat, caring tonality and a soft, easy, caring tempo and cadence. Hopefully, these simple scripts for phone calls and text messages will help you and your team facilitate these conversations more naturally to get more prospective patients scheduled effortlessly.

If you get these first five components down, your practice is ready for growth. When we run marketing campaigns for you, you can be confident that your team is well trained to turn the leads generated into new patients. However, there is one more factor that many practices miss. It is, in my opinion, the single most crucial thing your front desk must do to schedule 100% more consultations or essentially double the conversion rate of leads to new patients. That one thing is speed to lead. In the next chapter, you'll learn why the busiest practices in the country are calling leads back within five minutes.

CHAPTER 6

A Team That Embodies 'Speed to Lead'

"Can growing my practice really be as easy as calling leads back faster?"

I really can't harp on this enough. YES! When you have the other components in this book in place, all you have to do is make sure that your front desk calls every lead back within five minutes. That's it. It is that simple. Now is it easy? No, it's not. That's why you want to read the next few chapters very carefully. I will tell you exactly what to do so your scheduling coordinators never miss an opportunity to schedule a viable lead for their free consultation.

You must have a process in place for following up with prospective patients. Leads are most likely coming to you from various sources, such as calls and voicemails, form submissions on your website, or social media messages, comments, and campaigns. You have to think about how much time you have before these leads go cold. Most of the time, it's pretty quick.

Did you know that lead conversions are 391% higher if you call within one minute of an online inquiry (Velocify, 2012)? Studies show that when you call a lead back in five minutes versus thirty minutes, the odds of contacting a lead drop one hundred times with the long call-back period. They also show that the odds of qualifying that lead in the five-minute call-back period are twenty-one times higher than with the thirty-minute timeframe (Harvard Business Review, 2011). You may be missing out on dozens of leads per day just because you aren't getting to them quick enough–and it may be costing you millions.

It may sound impractical, but this call-back speed isn't impossible to achieve. Your front desk and scheduling team can do it with the right processes, people, and tools. And it can make all the difference between spending thousands on marketing for no results or blowing your Return on Investment (ROI) through the roof.

Digital Leads

Here's what you need to know about digital leads: they're just people sitting in front of their computers and phones, inquiring about products and services and hoping for instant gratification. Let's imagine this scenario. After brushing his teeth on a Tuesday morning, John looks in the mirror and thinks, *Ugh, my teeth have shifted. I should have worn my retainer.* He decides he's interested in Invisalign since he doesn't want to wear braces again as an adult. So, he walks to his desk, opens his computer, and begins searching for orthodontists in his area. He comes across your website. *Looks professional,* he thinks to himself, so he requests a free consultation. "Someone will get in touch with you shortly!" he reads on the screen.

John continues to research other practices in his area. After submitting a couple of requests for a free consultation, he comes across Smith Orthodontics. *All right, let's try this one, too.* He finds the 'request a free consultation' tab, inputs his information, and clicks send. As he's closing his laptop, his phone rings one minute later. "Hello! Is this John?" "Yes, hi." "Hi! This is Jan from Smith Orthodontics." Shocked, John replies, "WOW, that was fast. Hi!" And the consultation is booked. Thirty minutes later, John receives a follow-up from your practice. Unfortunately, he is no longer interested and turns down the appointment.

John's scenario gives us a glimpse of consumer behavior and the realities of today's world. With everything accessible at the click of a button, we aren't interested in waiting anymore. We will give our attention to the service that will gratify our needs quickly (think of our obsession with same-day shipping with Amazon Prime). It doesn't matter that he previously requested a consultation with you. He is unaware of your practice and your brand. He's not emotionally invested in you. Other practices provide the same treatment, so why should yours stand out? John doesn't appreciate the differences between competitors. He just wants Invisalign, and multiple places can offer it. But right now, Smith Orthodontics has his business because they responded immediately.

There are a few simple methods you can teach your team to get leads scheduled so this doesn't happen to you, such as the 5x6 method, the 72-hour rule, and virtual consultations, and using these methods can put you in the top 1% of successful practices.

The 5x6 Method

Train your front desk team to use the 5x6 method: they should contact every digital lead within five minutes of submitting a request and continue to follow up a minimum of six times. To ensure your leads don't slip through the cracks, they can use multiple channels to do this, such as by phone, text message, or email. A Harvard Business Review Study (2011) of 15,000 digital leads concluded that your chances of reaching a digital lead decrease by 900% if you don't respond within the first five minutes. However, you can boost your chances of contacting a lead to nearly 90% just by trying to contact them six times. If you hold your team accountable for this, you will see a noticeable improvement in your treatment coordinator's schedule.

The 72-Hour Rule

From the moment your lead confirms that they want a consultation, you should be able to book them onto your schedule within seventy-two hours. You have to schedule the patient as soon as possible, or they may just as easily use another competitor's services simply because they found an opening sooner than the appointment they booked with you. If your lead is scheduled within this seventy-two-hour window, their odds of no-showing decrease dramatically.

As we mentioned earlier, people like to be provided with quick services and don't want to wait for the things they think they should have right now. If your treatment coordinator's schedule is fully booked, let the patient know that the day is pretty busy, but you will try to squeeze them into the schedule. "It is best practice to leave one or two prime spots a day open to be scheduled quickly," says Alyx. Your leads may have waited weeks, months, or even years to have the courage to reach out to you finally. If you don't treat them like an urgent priority, they'll find someone else who does. By implementing the 72-hour rule, you'll see a significant increase in the number of starts, a considerable reduction in no-shows, and many more happy patients.

Virtual Consults

If you can't fit them in within seventy-two hours, always suggest a virtual consult instead. You must be thinking, virtual consults will only bring in low-quality leads–these people won't be serious about treatment, or virtual consults are just an extra step. You're wrong! The industry has found that virtual consults are helping doctors reach the ideal patients who have the budget to start treatment right away. These patients are working professionals who value efficiency over everything else since time is their most valuable resource. A virtual consult saves them another trip into the office, making it a more seamless process to get started. But it can also be beneficial for students with busy schedules or anyone who cannot make it in person for numerous reasons (i.e., a global pandemic that shut down the world for two years). The virtual appointment is the easiest option to get leads scheduled within seventy-two hours. If you are booked out for weeks, use this to your advantage. If your patient says they can't come in within the next few days, with platforms like SmileSnap, Rhinogram, and Clear-PG, it's easier than ever to offer these appointments. If you don't, then your competitors will.

Alyx knows the importance of getting in touch with leads quickly, so she has a few processes in place for her team to make sure they get them scheduled ASAP:

> *"My team knows that we need to get these leads the minute they come in, but obviously that's not always*

possible if they call on a Friday night when everyone has left the office. But they know that they must contact them first thing Monday morning and try to get them in for a same-day start. And if that isn't possible, they should suggest a virtual consult and highlight that they don't need to leave their house; they just need an internet connection. We give patients options so they know we're working with their schedules."

In a world where everything is accessible at the touch of a button, you have to act quickly when trying to get leads scheduled. They will just receive the same services somewhere else if you don't. If you're using these simple methods and teaching them to your front desk and scheduling team, there's no reason why any leads should be unacknowledged or missed. The numbers speak for themselves.

Of course, it's one thing to train your team on procedures and protocols and another thing that they follow through on performing the task exactly right every time. We aren't robots, and it is human nature to take shortcuts or delete things that seem boring or redundant. Unfortunately, what our brains deem unnecessary can often be the step that makes or breaks closing a lead. As we have seen throughout this book, the little things make a big difference in turning a lead into a patient and can add up to a million dollars to your bottom line. How do you make sure this is not happening in your practice? The answer is accountability, which we detail in the next chapter.

CHAPTER 7

A Team That is Accountable

Okay, you've taught your team the 5x6 method and the 72-hour rule and encouraged them to book virtual consults. Now what? How do you know they're doing all these things? When so many things are going on throughout the day, it can get tricky to determine if your employees are doing what they say. It's not enough to believe your team will do something just by asking them to do it. If you're not following up with them, critical steps and valuable leads will probably slip through the cracks now and then, or maybe consistently.

If you want consistent growth, you must know how your team follows up with each lead. If your team isn't following the same procedures every time, your efforts won't be nearly as effective; your growth may slow down or even come to a screeching halt. Most of the time, the proof is in the pudding, and you need to uncover that proof somehow. We can help you with that. The Secret Shop Report Card by PracticeBeacon ensures your team uses the proper follow-up procedures for every lead and holds them accountable for it.

The Secret Shop Report Card

Do you even know how many calls you got last week or last month? How many outbound calls were missed? How many leads were called or scheduled? Not paying attention to these questions can cost your business thousands of dollars each day. With the Secret Shop Report Card, you will be able to discover your team's accurate response times by providing a score for each interaction with a lead. Secret shops will occur online each month, and we will report back to you with their response times so you can hold them accountable.

Let's take a look at a few examples of report cards we've done on the practices we work with:

Example 1:

HIP

Secret Shop Report Card

Location Name:

Submission Date: Nov 17, 2021, 8:28 am CST

Report Generated On: Dec 4, 2021, 1:14 pm CST

Lead Name:

Lead Phone#:

Lead Email:

Total Score

17%

Results

PHONE CALLS

Suggested Process	Pass/Fail	Target Time To Call	How Quickly Was The Call Made	Voicemail
1st Call Within 05 Mins	⊗	05 mins	08 hrs:43 mins	✓
2nd Call Within 02 Hrs:00 Mins	⊗	02 hrs:00 mins	25 hrs:04 mins	⊗
3rd Call Within 25 Hrs:00 Mins	⊗	25 hrs:00 mins	25 hrs:54 mins	⊗

Touchpoints Summary

SMS	Calls	Voicemails	Email	Touchpoints
5	7	2	0	14

Before we go over the results, let's break down the Secret Shop Report Card features. On the top left corner, you will see the location name, the date when the report card was submitted, the date when the report card was generated, and the lead's name, phone number, and email. You will see a percentage of the total score in the top right corner, the results breakdown in the middle, and the touchpoints summary from start to finish at the bottom. This includes SMS [text messages], phone calls, voicemails, emails, and the combined total score of these touchpoints.

In this first example, the employee scored a 17% for their follow-up efforts with this lead. It took them almost 9 hours for the initial call and 25 hours for the second and third follow-up calls. They only left a voicemail after the initial call but failed to do so during the second and third calls. Their total touchpoints were pretty high at 14, so it is safe to say that the lead was no longer interested in continuing with the conversation.

Example 2:

HIP

Secret Shop Report Card

Location Name:

Submission Date: Mar 7, 2022, 1:08 pm CST

Report Generated On: Mar 17, 2022, 9:09 am CDT

Lead Name:

Lead Phone#:

Lead Email:

Total Score

33%

Results

PHONE CALLS

Suggested Process	Pass/Fail	Target Time To Call	How Quickly Was The Call Made	Voicemail
1st Call Within 05 Mins	✓	05 mins	03 mins	✗
2nd Call Within 02 Hrs:00 Mins	✗	02 hrs:00 mins	73 hrs:06 mins	✓
3rd Call Within 25 Hrs:00 Mins	✗	25 hrs:00 mins	No Call	✗

Touchpoints Summary

SMS	Calls	Voicemail	Email	Touchpoints
8	2	1	0	11

The scheduling coordinator scored slightly higher at 33% in the second example. They called the lead back in 3 minutes, but it took them 73 hours for a second call when it should have taken 2 hours, and they didn't even bother to call a third time. They only left one voicemail during the second attempt. The total touchpoints were fairly good as the scheduling coordinator sent many text messages, but they should have put more effort into the phone calls.

Example 3:

HIP

Secret Shop Report Card

Location Name:

Submission Date: Mar 15, 2022, 2:25 pm EDT

Report Generated On: Mar 28, 2022, 9:16 am EDT

Lead Name:

Lead Phone#:

Lead Email:

Total Score

83%

Results

PHONE CALLS

Suggested Process	Pass/Fail	Target Time To Call	How Quickly Was The Call Made	Voicemail
1st Call Within 05 Mins	✓	05 mins	00 mins	✓
2nd Call Within 02 Hrs:00 Mins	✗	02 hrs:00 mins	04 hrs:49 mins	✓
3rd Call Within 25 Hrs:00 Mins	✓	25 hrs:00 mins	19 hrs:44 mins	✓

Touchpoints Summary

SMS	Calls	Voicemails	Email	Touchpoints
8	3	3	0	14

In the third example, the scheduling coordinator did an excellent job with the follow-up, scoring an 83% with this lead. The first call took place right away, which is amazing, but it took them almost 5 hours to make the second call. If they got that second call down to 2 hours, they would have received a 100% score. The scheduling coordinator also left a voicemail after all three rings and had very high touchpoints with the lead, as they also sent numerous text messages as reminders. This is what needs to be done every single time for scheduling coordinators to receive 100% secret shop report card scores when following up with leads.

I think it would be beneficial to show your employees the results of their secret shop report card. These results will enable them to see where they need to improve and motivate them to do better next time around. However, you shouldn't do this to shame them or make them feel bad about themselves.

What if my employee consistently produces poor results?

If you have had multiple coaching conversations with an employee who is still delivering poor results, it may be time to consider alternative options. Before you make any drastic decisions, take the time to sit down with your employee to find out what is preventing them from achieving their goals and targets. There can be numerous reasons why their performance may be dwindling. Maybe it's a personal or a work-related issue? Perhaps they need to be re-trained on specific processes and procedures? Perhaps they have difficulty keeping up with the volume of leads coming in and require more help?

As mentioned earlier in this book, you need to make sure your team is motivated to serve your patients and determined to achieve the goals set out for the practice. Whatever it may be, it is essential to have a one-on-one conversation with them to determine where they need support. But you must also do your part to listen and make the necessary changes to enable them to succeed. If these efforts still result in poor performance based on these report cards, it may be time to let the employee go.

Holding your team accountable with the Secret Shop Report Card by PracticeBeacon, will help your team make daily improvements to deliver the highest standard of service that your patients deserve. In the next chapter, you will learn more about what PracticeBeacon has to offer your practice, but if you are interested in just testing out our Secret Shop tool before committing to our services, contact us to try it out!

CHAPTER **8**

A Team That Succeeds With Tracking and Transparency

Jan at Smith Orthodontics seems to have everything figured out. She's scheduling around 110 leads per month by reaching out to every lead as soon as the request comes through her computer. She's upbeat, ready to work, and always up for a challenge. She knows her day will run smoothly, so she doesn't sweat the small stuff. Smith Orthodontics consistently has the best secret shop scores every month in Florida. Is that just because of Jan? It partially is. But Lori is also scheduling approximately 100 leads per month. And Kim is scheduling around 90 leads per month. That's about 300 leads a month for Smith Orthodontics.

Smith Orthodontics reached out to us three years ago to grow their practice. They started with annual revenue of two million dollars, and today, they produce over eight million dollars in revenue annually and currently have three locations in the state. Jan, Lori, and Kim didn't just devote themselves to working 24/7 to make that growth possible. They also didn't wish upon a star to make it happen. Instead, Smith Orthodontics realized they needed one crucial element in their practice to bring that goal to life: an automated system.

How can automation help you?

There are some things that you just can't expect your front desk team to do every time, such as contacting a lead within five minutes at 2:00 am on a Tuesday. There are other things that automation can do more efficiently, like sending three emails, three text messages, and three phone calls to every new lead within twenty-four hours of first contact. For tracking and transparency to be a smooth and straightforward action, PracticeBeacon (PB) can be utilized to make your front desk and scheduling team work efficiently without overwhelming them. In the previous chapter, you discovered how secret shop report cards would help you hold your team accountable. So, now that you have a taste of one function of PB that will help your follow-up process, let's get into the bulk of what PB is and why it is essential for the growth of your practice.

What is PracticeBeacon?

For your business to grow exponentially, the tracking

process is crucial. PracticeBeacon (PB) is our proprietary CRM software that we created to help you automate follow-ups, convert more leads, and see how much money you are making from your digital advertisements. PB is packed with features that will automate and optimize your lead management to make tracking an effortless process. It will help boost your team's effectiveness and efficiency by assisting them in booking more appointments, reducing no-shows, and cutting out time-wasting tasks. They will be able to fill your calendar consistently without feeling overwhelmed, automate critical new patient interactions to help them schedule more consults, and see the new patient communication clearer than ever. Moreover, you will understand if the money you're spending on marketing is bringing you new patients and watch all of your marketing channels to know which ones are making you the most money.

What does that look like?

PB will automatically send your prospective patient's information, so you never have to worry about it being missed or forgotten. Here's what it looks like:

- Text/email #1 will auto-send immediately after the initial conversation.
    - You only need to manually respond if the patient replies to the text or email within 24 hours.
- Text/email #2 will auto-send the following day.

- Text/email #3 will auto-send 48 hours after opting.

Having several touchpoints with a new lead is paramount. Even though this automation is set up as a catch-all, phone calls are essential for setting the appointment. Your team can utilize the phone call function in PB if they:

- Check if the patient responded to the automation.
    - If they haven't, your team knows to call the new prospect within 5 minutes, ideally 1 minute.
- Call again after 2 hours.
- Make the third call within 24 hours of opt-in.

If the prospective patient doesn't schedule (or respond), then PracticeBeacon will continue to send a "nurture" sequence for 30 days. This is a series of texts and emails. We also recommend calling once a week to check in with the opportunity.

How can PB help your practice?

Ultimately, we made PB as simple as possible so that your day-to-day tasks can be as streamlined as a busy office demands. Your team will be able to send text and email automation, engage in two-way text messaging, send and receive emails, record phone calls, and efficiently contribute to social messaging. You will be able to optimize your front desk by scheduling online, sending appointment reminders, providing curbside check-ins, and following up with prospects via the chat widget, all in one convenient place! You will also be able to see what you earn by analyzing your return on investment in real-time and discover the source of your new patients, such as from Facebook, Google, referrals, etc.

Does my front desk team need to know everything on PB?

No! Your front desk will only need to pay attention to a few functions in PB. The conversations and opportunities tabs are where they will spend most of their time for day-to-day tasks, but they will also have access to the training portal and FAQs section.

Conversations

The conversations tab will help your team manage phone calls, voicemails, text messages, emails, and follow-up with new leads. It will allow your team to insert notes on patient files and set up tasks and reminders to update patients instantaneously. It will save your team time and energy by providing seamless communication from the touch of a button without even needing to dial the phone.

Opportunities

The opportunities tab is the pipeline where all new leads come in. Your team will be able to see prospective patients who have responded to your reactivation campaigns and requested a free consultation, keeping all of your leads in one accessible program. PB's opportunities feature will also allow your team to:

- Track how many times they have manually reached out to a prospective patient and keep track of the voicemails sent to them.
- View all scheduled appointments.
- See how many prospective patients have pending treatments.
- Determine patients who are not ready to start treatment and keep them under observation until treatment can begin.
- Put patients who have started treatment in a single column to keep them organized and easy to track.

Training Portal

The training portal will help new users of PB learn and view step-by-step procedure modules to help navigate the program and its associated functions. These training videos will help your team:

- Determine how and when prospective patients

receive communication from PB after they opt-in to your offer, how to use the Contact list within PracticeBeacon, including adding a contact, searching for a connection, using smart lists, and more.

- Use 'Tasks' to assign items and set due dates for team members.
- View assigned tasks from the Dashboard and sort tasks by ascending and descending.
- Make a call using PB and track call reports.
- Change the contact and opportunity names.
- Find script templates to structure specific calls, emails, and text messages.
- Manage the schedule columns and use their calendar.

FAQs

Finally, if there are any uncertainties, your team will also have access to basic FAQs with videos for areas where they might get stuck and need additional support, such as:

- What is a reactivation campaign?
- How do tracking numbers and emails work?
- How to set up notifications on a Mac?

- How to set up notifications on a PC?

If your team has additional questions that have not already been addressed in the training portal or FAQs section, feel free to contact us directly. We will consistently add more training and FAQs to PB based on your feedback and comments for future use and reference!

Providing Feedback via PB

We've discussed how providing feedback to your team is essential if you want to see growth happen. I understand that it's hard to check in on your team to make sure they're doing everything the way you want them to. That's why we created a function on PB that allows us to track your team's conversations to see if they're following the right processes, and we provide them with feedback on how they can improve. Simple, right? You don't have to do anything. We'll do it for you and fill you in on the results.

We will create and invite you to your own Google Doc where we will leave comments (which can be written notes, screenshots, sound clips, etc.) about what we've observed in both text message exchanges and recorded phone calls between leads and scheduling coordinators. We will highlight the lead's name, a note of what happened, the status of the lead, and HIP's recommendation for future interactions. This is a great way to hold your team accountable for the follow-up process while also ensuring that great service is continually being provided to patients via phone call or text message. Beyond the Google Doc, we will also periodically set up live training calls with your team. We also offer a consulting package with weekly group calls where we continue to drill best practices. Lastly, if things are clicking, we have a 4-week course that is hyper-focused on getting your schedulers to where they need to be regarding lead management and the new patient experience.

Here are a few examples to show you what this feedback document looks like:

****Please note, the names have been changed to protect the individual's privacy.***

Example 1 [Text Message]:

Name: Tim Smalls

Notes: No notes made in PB

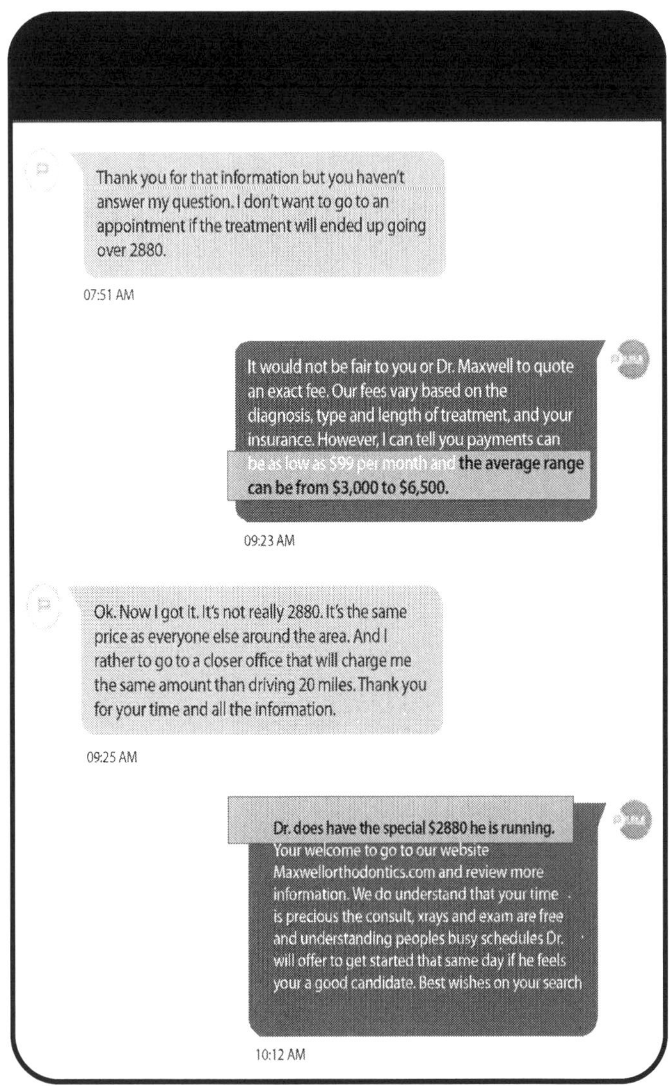

Status in PB: Lost

HIP recommendation: It seems Jessica (the scheduler) was not aware of the special until the end of the conversation. She should have pitched a virtual consult after hearing that the prospective patient is 20-miles away! Just lost $2,800.00 for this limited treatment case. Let's present convenience and excellent service.

Example 2 (Phone Call):

Name: Jane Jones

Note in PB: When Jane asked what the cost of treatment was, I told her that every person's case is different, so I won't be able to tell her the cost of treatment over the phone and that she needs to come in for a consultation. She got upset and said that if she couldn't get the full cost, she isn't interested in scheduling.

Status in PB: Lost

HIP recommendation: Call PB leads in PB. This way, we can hear the call. I'm really interested to see how fees were presented here. You need to give an average! Don't ever lead with a total price. That will "sticker shock" the prospect. Instead, tell them how affordable you've made it. "While we have to see you....the average is $X down and as low as $99/mo..."

Example 3 (Text Message):

Name: Lisa Maniscola
Notes: No notes made in PB

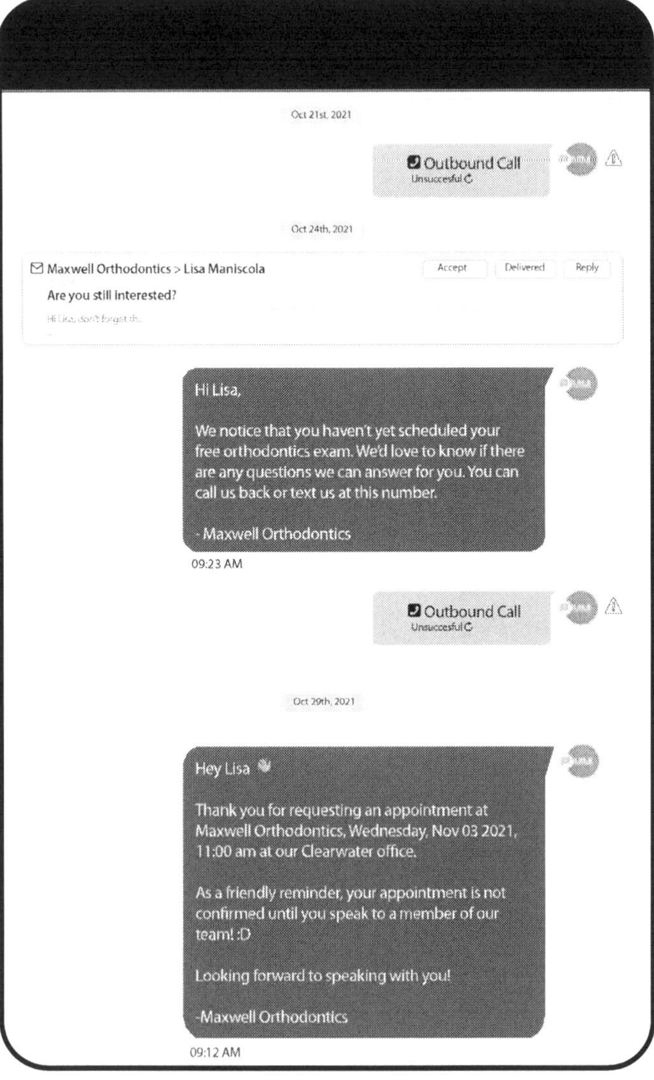

Status in PB: Open (and marked Interested)

HIP recommendation: She reached out twice, from a Facebook ad AND scheduled online. No notes and no follow-up. The "outbound call unsuccessful" alert shows that PB attempted to connect the office with the patient and the front desk declined the call. She was definitely interested. How many people have become interested and then just went cold due to not keeping them warm with proper follow-up?

In the first two examples, the leads went cold because there were miscommunications about fees and pricing from the scheduling coordinator. In the last example, the scheduling coordinator didn't follow up at all, even though the lead was interested.

There are a few takeaways to note from these examples:

- Make sure your team is aware of any new promotions to relay information to prospective patients accurately.
- For regular pricing and fee information, provide an average so they have some information to work with, even if you can't provide the total cost.
- Follow up with text messages, phone calls, and always leave notes.
- Never let the lead go cold.

Keep Your Leads on Your Radar

As you can see by the examples, leads can go cold pretty quickly when your team isn't trained properly, and you don't have the right systems in place. Your team has to stay on top of it the minute they come through your pipeline. So, I'm giving you four magic rules you can use with your team when following up with leads to make sure small errors don't get in the way of getting them scheduled:

1. You should send "love touches" whenever possible. A "love touch" just means checking in on prospective patients to see how they're doing and if they've given any thought to a consultation or treatment.
2. You should consistently WOW them with great service. Don't chase them away with a poor attitude or neglect to provide them with essential information. Leads will stick around if you give them a reason to.
3. The ball should always be left in their court, not yours. Their messages to you should NEVER be left unanswered. You should always have the last word in, then follow up if they don't respond.
4. Always keep the lead warm! Follow up, follow up, love touch, follow up!

If you remember to follow these four simple rules when conducting your follow-up process, there shouldn't be any reason for leads to go cold.

Accountability is one attribute that sets the most successful practices apart from the mediocre ones. Still, it does not mean that you have to act like a big brother, constantly policing your teams' every move. The top producing practices have a great deal of concern for the well-being of their team members. They want the job to be enjoyable and are concerned when things get too busy for the team to handle. That is why a few cutting-edge practices have made the leap to separating the job of answering the phones and scheduling appointments from greeting patients and directing office flow.

In the nation's most successful orthodontic practices, you will most likely find a call center that handles all incoming calls, leads, and scheduling coordination. We like to call this a "patient care center" because when the schedule coordinators are well trained, the level of service sets the stage for the WOW experience the patient can expect when they come to the office. In the following chapter, we will dive into how simple setting up a patient care center in your practice could be.

CHAPTER 9

A Team That Benefits From the Patient Care Center

I want you to put yourself in your patients' shoes and walk into your practice to check in for your first appointment. The front desk team member is on the phone and raises her hand to you with the "one-second gesture." She appears to be speaking to a disgruntled patient who can't find a time to bring in her son for his next visit. A patient, who has just finished an appointment, steps in line behind you to schedule their next appointment on their way out. The phones keep ringing, and everyone in the lobby can hear them. It's your first time here and now you're thinking, Great. Here we go again. Another doctor's office. I hope I don't have to come back here too often.

If the person at the desk was only focused on greeting people when they came in and rebooking those leaving, this situation could have been avoided. The solution is a call center or patient care center, as we like to call them. It can start with as few as two or three people, and you don't need a lot of space. Most importantly, you free up the front desk to provide the WOW service that your patients deserve.

Many orthodontists are opposed to the idea at first. They think of the typical stereotype of call centers outsourced to another country and feel that it is too impersonal for their practice. They fail to consider that their front desk team can't do everything at once and provide excellent service. Everyone wins by simply splitting the roles at the front desk to have people dedicated to greeting and rebooking patients and another set of people whose job is to handle incoming calls and provide a fantastic first impression of your practice to new leads.

Is there a correlation between the highest-grossing practices in the country and having a patient care center? Yes! When you separate calling and scheduling from greeting and patient care (check-in, scheduling future appointments, etc.), your patient experience improves, your team satisfaction improves, and your production doubles.

Happy Employees = Happy Patients

When you think about the service and the patient experience a patient care center would bring, you will add more value to your practice. You will let patients know that you care, that it's about them, not you, and they deserve your undivided attention. By ridding your front desk team of phone duty, they will be able to move more freely around the office, provide better service to patients, and ultimately allow them to feel less stress and pressure while at work. The same goes for your patient care center team. They will have one designated role throughout their workday, allowing them to quickly answer every call and get those important leads scheduled every time.

A patient care center is vital for practices that have multiple locations, and there is a need for a centralized team to handle the volume of calls for each location. If you want to see your practice grow from where it is currently to one that takes in multiple seven or eight figures of revenue every year, this is not a component you should overlook.

Julie loves the addition of the patient care center in her office:

> *"Everyone on our team, like the front desk, clinic admin, and doctors, understands the value of the patient care center. We're opening up a fourth location now, so we had to add a centralized team that handles all phone calls. We opened it up at the beginning of the pandemic and it's been the best thing for our practice. The patient care center took a lot of tasks away from the front desk. Since we have such a high volume of leads every day, the team can now focus on just answering the phones.*

And the people at the front desk now have more time to focus on the people in the office. It not only has made things easier to manage, but it has also made us better at teamwork. When one person needs help, another person can easily step in because that person is no longer bombarded with so many tasks. And I have to say, we can feel it now when the designated patient care center person isn't there. It's hectic. We're definitely really excited to see them when they walk through the doors."

Alyx has seen dramatic improvements in her patient's experiences:

"The patient care center has really taken the pressure off our front desk team. By creating an area in the practice that's solely for answering phone calls, we've been able to make a huge difference in our patients' experiences, in the office and on the phone. We've recently had a patient ask, "where's the person I talked to on the phone??" because they just wanted to say hi and thank them for their awesome attitude and service. So many patients come in and say that we've made their day. We even had a patient send flowers to a girl working in our patient care center just because she went above and beyond and made her life easier. It's just really cool to see that kind of reaction."

What if I can't afford it?

If you're still concerned about the cost of bringing on and paying new employees to fill patient care center positions, then let me paint you a picture. You've decided to set one up in your practice and hired two people to fill those roles. You're paying a salary of $50,000.00 for each employee. You trained them well with the materials we've provided you, and so far, they're doing a great job speaking with patients. Your front desk team is making a great impression on the patients in the office, and they seem happier since they aren't distracted by constant phone calls throughout the day. They're caring for your existing patients and keeping them happy. Your patient care center answers 98% of all inbound phone calls, and they've scheduled 50 leads each for new patient consultations within the last month. Let's fast forward to a year from now, and this trend has continued. Does an additional $100,000.00 matter to you now that you've tripled your revenue from last year? Probably not.

We encourage our biggest practices to put a patient care center in place if they have not already. We recommend it to practices around the two to three million dollar mark. It can be as simple as moving the person answering the phones to another room and respecting how busy she is scheduling new patients, but it is not for everyone. Some people simply cannot wrap their heads around the fact that it is a call center and believe it is too impersonal for their practice. That's okay. You can still be successful and grow without one, but I consider it a best practice among the nation's fastest-growing orthodontic practices. In the next chapter, we'll share some other best practices that you can use to elevate your team and office.

CHAPTER 10

A Team That Understands the Best Practices For Growth

As we wrap up the "Ten Components of the Front Desk of Your Dreams", I want to finish by sharing some best practices to keep your team and practice growing. I realize that this is a work in progress for all teams striving for excellence. At this point, it must be clear that being well-trained in processes and procedures and performing them flawlessly every time is the key to success.

I consider separating your front desk into the patient care center and front desk a pro move and a best practice for practices that want to experience next-level growth. Again, this is not for everyone, and I've seen practices grow very well without doing this.

Julie and her team have figured out the ground rules they have to follow to make sure the front desk and patient care center teams interact efficiently throughout the day:

"Over the last few years, we've figured out how to navigate having a call center in our office. We've learned that this is their designated time to work, so we can't interrupt them all of the time by walking in. When they first started, it was easy to drop off a document or stop by to have a chat. But then we realized that wasn't sustainable since they receive such a high volume of calls every day. When we need to talk now, we usually communicate via email so we at least have a record of everything we've discussed, and we can reference it later."

Technology

Set your front desk and patient care center teams up with functioning and up-to-date computer software to handle applications and programs. If you use PraticeBeacon or another CRM system, your phone calls, emails, and text messages come directly from the software, so make sure you have internet with a strong enough bandwidth and signal to keep up with the demand. If your internet connection is poor, you will most likely miss out on opportunities.

Wireless headsets are an excellent option for practices with a patient care team and those with front desk teams who do it all. They allow your team to keep their hands free to multitask, talk on the phone, type on their keyboard, write on their note pads, or even walk to another clinic area, all while getting the patient scheduled. It is ultimately the key to success and the only way to not kill your neck from holding a phone to your ear all day.

I timed patient interactions performed by a scheduling coordinator to compare the length of calls using a phone to those using a wireless headset. Consistently, bookings made using the phone took an average of six minutes, while the appointments scheduled using a headset took an average of three minutes. Headsets effectively cut the time it takes to make a booking in half.

Alyx and her team have only had positive experiences after implementing wireless headsets in their patient care center:

> *"Headsets have been a game-changer for us. The patient care center team loves it. We never had them before when we just had a front desk area. Now that we have a patient care center, all the scheduling coordinators have a wireless headset. And it's great because I'll notice some of the team members walking around the office while on the call with a patient as they're grabbing a new payment form in another area. But they can still keep talking to them instead of putting them on hold. We're really trying to minimize hold times; if we can prevent it, we will. So the headsets have been really helping us achieve that."*

Resources

As we now know, there's a lot to remember in the front desk and scheduling coordinator role. There are many steps to make this process perfect, and sometimes it's hard to remember everything during an interaction. We miss things sometimes; we're only human. That's why it is essential to provide the necessary resources to your team, whether instructions on how to use

PracticeBeacon, tips about tonality and tempo to keep in mind, or even scripts to help facilitate a smooth conversation while getting the correct information. Set your teams up for success so that they can deliver in return! Your team will be thankful to have these resources at their disposal, which will take the pressure off them if they forget the small details.

Beverly finds the day-to-day relatively easy when there are resources to use when she's speaking with leads all day:

> *"Sometimes it's helpful to have a checklist of everything I need to do within the day at my desk. I also have the simple scripts I can pull from when interacting with a new lead or booking new patient consults. I talk to many people throughout the day, so it's easy to skip a step if you aren't thinking about all the steps involved. Having an outline of everything I need to go over readily accessible ensures I never miss something, and the patient can give me all their information within that one short phone call."*

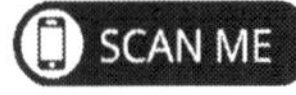

To access our PracticeBeacon Quick Guide please scan this QR Code.

SCAN ME

To watch a quick 10-minute video outlining the fundamentals you need for the perfect front desk, scan this QR code.

How much do you want to grow?

At this point, we've given you a few tips and tricks to work with to take on those leads quickly. You're probably wondering HOW impactful these strategies are. I can assure you, it's all you need to do to see changes in your team's work ethic and your annual production. But you may want to ask yourself: how much do I really want to grow? Maybe you're comfortable remaining as a one-location practice with around $1,000,000.00 in annual revenue and enjoy having a small team, but you want to make sure your schedules are consistently staying filled. Maybe you're looking to add more departments and teams to your one location so you can take on more patients and grow your annual revenue. Or perhaps you're looking to open multiple locations throughout your state or even the country and build various teams.

Whatever your goals are, you need to have a plan, and you need to have support. I've provided you with some charts to help you visualize what different kinds of practices look like. Some practices only have one location and a few team members, while others have multiple locations and numerous departments and teams.Hopefully, these charts will enable you to envision where you'd like to see your practice grow or help you to determine which roles you'd like to add to your current practice to make it easier to manage.

Practice Organization Charts

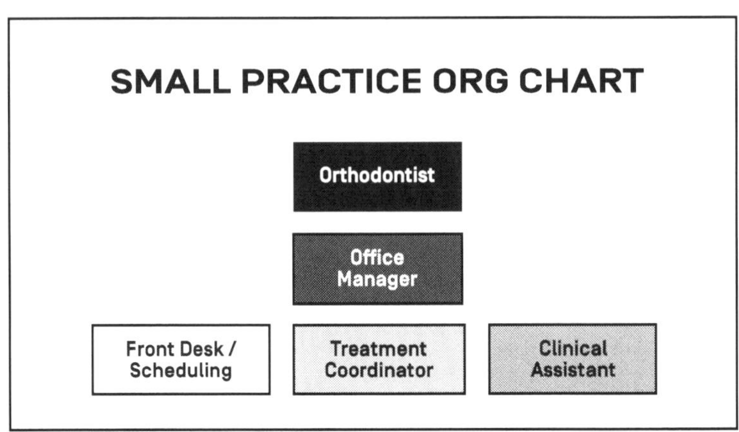

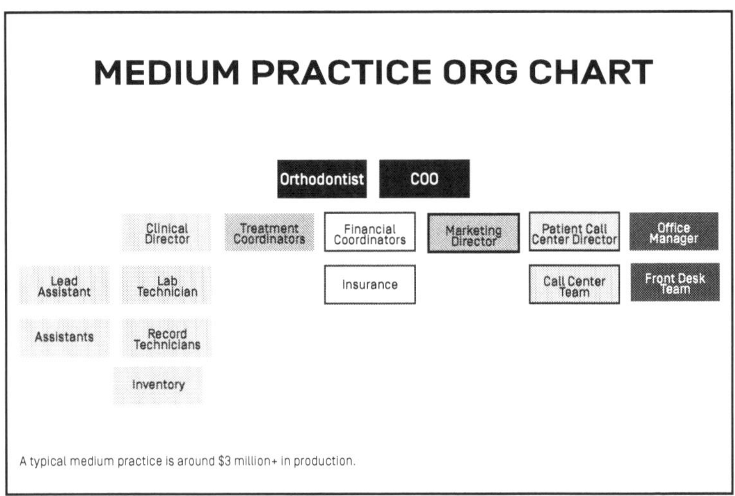

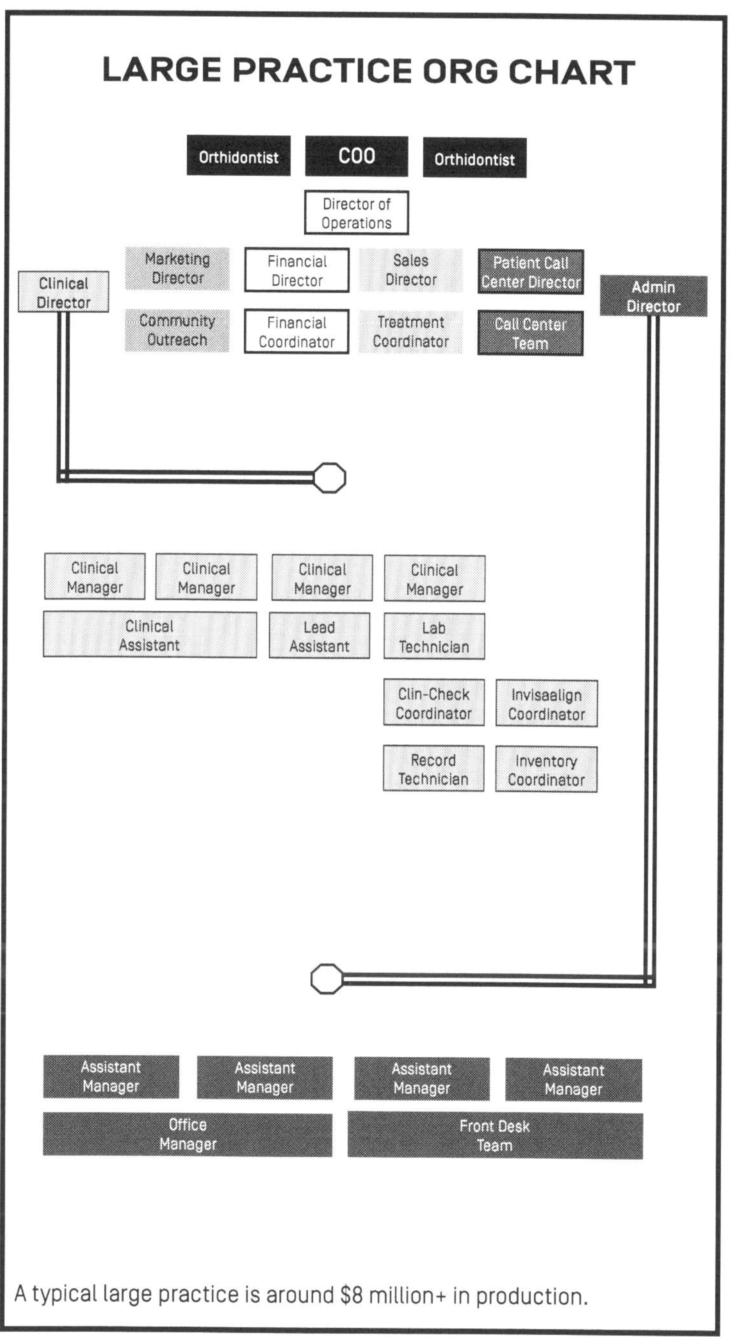
LARGE PRACTICE ORG CHART
Orthidontist
COO
Orthidontist
Director of Operations
Marketing Director
Financial Director
Sales Director
Patient Call Center Director
Clinical Director
Admin Director
Community Outreach
Financial Coordinator
Treatment Coordinator
Call Center Team
Clinical Manager
Clinical Manager
Clinical Manager
Clinical Manager
Clinical Assistant
Lead Assistant
Lab Technician
Clin-Check Coordinator
Invisaalign Coordinator
Record Technician
Inventory Coordinator
Assistant Manager
Assistant Manager
Assistant Manager
Assistant Manager
Office Manager
Front Desk Team
A typical large practice is around $8 million+ in production.

What does approximately a year of growth look like?

I'm going to provide you with some examples of what approximately one year of growth looks like by showcasing the ROIs of two practices we currently work with: Knecht Orthodontics and All Smiles Orthodontics. These examples demonstrate how all the components work together to produce bottom-line results when implemented correctly.

Knecht Orthodontics is an example of a small practice we're currently working with. They partnered with us two years ago when they were just a start-up, as they were interested in understanding the best practices for the practice from the get-go. After setting them up with PracticeBeacon and training their team on all of the components mentioned in this book, Knecht Orthodontics rose to the occasion and accomplished their goal in less than a year.

In October 2020, Knecht invested $48,150.00 into their practice [$34,650.00 in HIP consulting and $13,500.00 on advertisements]. By August 2021, their amount returned [the 61 leads who have started treatment] was $275,000, having gained $226,850 in investments and increased their ROI by 471% in less than 10 months. This isn't total production; it's just from our framework [basically, digital leads turning into new patients]. And those are just from patients who have started treatment.

To determine Knecht's Estimated Potential Production, we calculate the revenue generated when every lead that starts completes their treatment plan. As the leads follow through, the potential revenue gained is what the new patient pays during their treatment. So, the additional amount returned would be $61,000.00, bringing their total investment gain to $561,850.00 and an ROI of 1,166.87%. This was in 2020, and as previously mentioned, Dr. Knecht produced well over a million dollars in her first full year opened (2021) and was able to transition into her start-up full-time, which was a huge milestone!

Remember All Smiles Orthodontics? I showed you their ROI Calculation at the beginning of this book. Don't worry, you don't have to turn back to find it. We'll go over it again here. All Smiles Orthodontics is an example of a large practice we're currently working with. Here is a breakdown of All Smile's ROI, starting from May 2020 to August 2021, based on 268 completed patient treatments:

- An initial investment of $171,500.00.
- A return amount of $1,000,000.00.
- An investment gain of $828,500.00.
- An ROI of 483.09%.

And if they were to get all pending leads to complete their treatment today, their Estimated Potential Production would be an additional $4,000,000.00 to their amount returned, bringing their total investment gain to $4,228,500.00 and an ROI of 2,465.60%. Again, this isn't their entire production. We are just sharing their growth from our framework, and this is all tracked in PracticeBeacon.

The numbers don't lie. Both Knecht and All Smiles Orthodontics decided to invest in their practices and have since reaped the rewards by pulling in hundreds of thousands to millions of dollars worth of investment gains in less than a year. This is possible when you implement the ten components I've discussed in this book. I hope you and your team take them to heart and implement them into your practice so you can enjoy results like this, too.

Conclusion

When I was fifteen years old, I really wanted a job. My parents were great, but they only paid for the basics I needed to stay alive, and hey, I NEEDED cool clothes, burgers, and video games. When I got hired at Chick-fil-A, the manager told me that they hired me because they were sick of me coming back every week, submitting another application, and tracking them down to ask if they were ready to hire me. I guess I intuitively grasped the concept of follow-up at that early age!

I wanted to work there because it was the only decent place to work that would teach me good skills and hired fifteen-year-olds. Chick-fil-A boasted about the quality of their people, and I didn't want to be around unmotivated people in a dead-end job.

Looking back, it was way more than just a job. That experience shaped who I am today and is coded in our DNA at HIP. They are known for their excellent customer service and leadership, and they run the quickest drive-through in the world. They have this phrase, "In the red," which means the orders have over five minutes of customers waiting. When that code is signaled, literally everyone (managers, janitors, and anyone else on the floor) comes running to get out of the red!

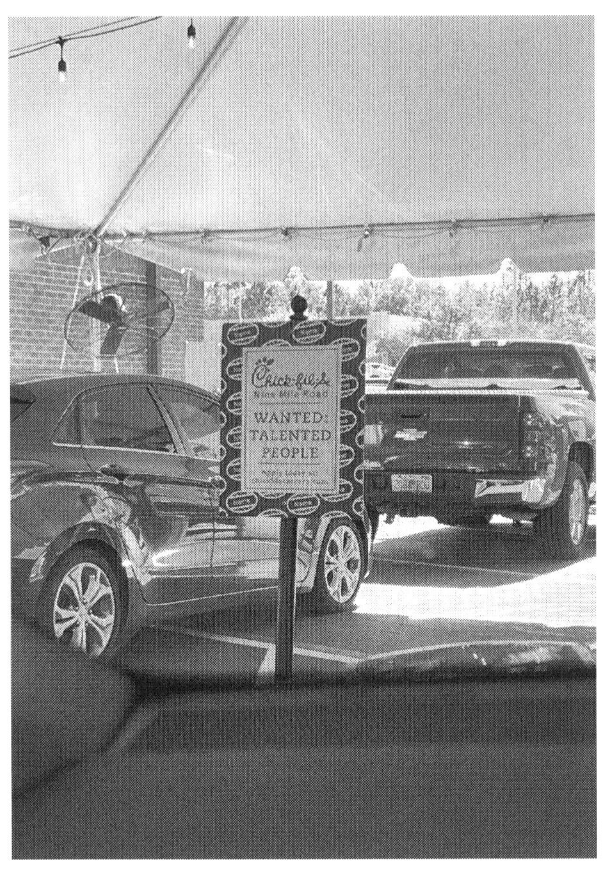

I really took to their training, and I loved learning about effective communication. They basically invented or brought back the saying, "my pleasure." In my opinion, this little phrase goes a long way and is leagues better than saying, "no problem" or "no worries." You could get written up for using the wrong language. After all, it is our pleasure to serve and never a problem or worry!

I was put in charge of their leadership program and distributed packets to all new employees with motivational training from Zig Ziglar and Jim Rohn. They had their own curriculum, as well. This was pre-framed with, "If for some reason our leadership program doesn't resonate with you, it's ok! There's another place out there for you." If new employees didn't move from a level 1 leader to a level 2 leader in 90 days, they were removed from the team.

Fast forward a decade and a bit, when I started doing marketing for orthodontists, it did not take me long to recognize that their front desks were the biggest opportunity for their growth and success. Going to check-in at the front desk is kind of like going up to the counter at Chick-fil-A to order some chicken nuggets and waffle fries. At Chick-fil-A, you get exactly what you want fast AND the person serving you makes your day. At the orthodontist... well let's just say lots of practices missed the mark. It just killed me to watch them spend thousands of dollars a month on marketing to flush it down the toilet due to lousy customer service, poor lead management, and terrible sales processes.

I created the "Ten Components of the Front Desk of Your Dreams" to help you reap the benefits of every lesson I learned from Chick-fil-A AND the top orthodontics practices across the country that we have the privilege of partnering with. I hope you see many opportunities to up-level your team, improve your patient experience, and move toward the practice you envision.

The way I see it, there are three key takeaways in this book:

1. The front desk is the most important and most overlooked role in the orthodontic practice.
2. The person who has first contact with new leads has the most critical job in your clinic.
3. If your team responds to those leads faster with top-notch service, you will make way more money (and get to serve way more new patients).

Grasping these three concepts and getting them instilled in your team will transform your practice. And yes, it IS way easier said than done.

At HIP, my team and I work with orthodontic practices every day to put these components in place. We've made a documentary about the orthodontic practice transformations that we have enjoyed participating in. If you'd like to see it, please scan this QR code.

You'll be able to see what happens when we help a practice nail the four principles for orthodontic practice growth:

1. The orthodontist is a technician, not a manager (so hire a good one).
2. Training your team to follow the steps to convert every viable lead into a new patient (and there are no bad leads).
3. Marketing to attract the right leads.

4. Software that tracks your metrics and holds your team accountable for the goals you've set.

I invite you to take the first step in building the front desk of your dreams right now. Dr. Sarah Howle, an associate at Fishbein Orthodontics, says, "What gets inspected gets RESPECTED." Scan this QR code and get a secret shop done in your practice today.

SCAN ME

If you have any questions, comments, or success stories, please reach out! You can email me at luke@hipcreativeinc.com.

I wish you great success in your practice. Thank you for letting me share my vision for the amazing people who work at front desks worldwide.

Luke Infinger
March 2022

Made in the USA
Columbia, SC
17 February 2023

12503011R00078